MW00512351

MEMOIRS FROM CALIBRATED EYES

SANDY O.

ARBUCKLE PUBLISHING HOUSE

CONTENTS

*God made my Father and my Mother – I am a concoction of that union. I want to give thanks to God for constructing me and letting me use his ingredients for the betterment of others. I thank God that he did not make me shy, did not make me weak, and has instilled in me the ability to receive, learn, and output all the vowels, consonants, and 'E's that can be formed for his purposes. I owe everything to **Him**, and I mean everything. I am blessed!*

For information contact :
Arbuckle Publishing House
arbucklepublishinghouse.com

Written by Sandy O.
Published by Arbuckle Publishing House LLC
Cover by Arbuckle Publishing House
ISBN: 978-1-952255-39-7

Multiple Sclerosis ... more like Scultiple Mlerosis

Memoirs
From
Calibrated
Eyes

Sandy O.

MEMOIRS FROM CALIBRATED EYES

SANDY O.

APH | Arbuckle
Publishing House

1

SAY WHAT?!

JUNE 24

WHAT ON EARTH IS HAPPENING? Ahh!

I have *what?*

You've gotta be friggin' kidding me!

I have to get to the beginnings of this disgusting bombardment of chaos... The who/what/where/why & when of the saga must come out.

One thing you must know about me right away is that I don't lie. For me, *not* to say everything about what I've experienced with Multiple Sclerosis (MS) feels like lying, so I'm not going to do that. For all those feeling shoved in a cubbyhole and for the lives with no voice or say in their own world, I will be that voice in this book.

Let me hold your embarrassment because I am not embarrassed of what has happened to me. I'll say it again. This happened *to me*, I did not invite it in. I didn't do anything wrong! That's inevitably what people do once they get bad news, like a diagnosis of Multiple Sclerosis (MS). I certainly self-analyzed everything.

Did I bring this nightmare onto myself?

I know this – every single thing you keep a secret that's not your fault can become a weapon used against you. I make it a point never to hand anybody the knife to stab me with. In this book, you will hear things other people don't want to say out loud because... it's a *secret*, an embarrassing s e c r e t.

Bump that!

No symptoms will make me feel like I have to hide from the world...

Nope, not goin' to happen!

First things first, no one in my family has ever been diagnosed with MS. To center you on the map, it's the late 1980s and I have a very clear recollection of all the compounds I dealt with in my career. I remember one in particular that said it was linked to this disease. Because the MSDS (material safety data sheets) were not up front and center in the beginning of my career (that I recall), I later became the queen of understanding the innards of an MSDS and taught new people how to read them and take the listed precautions seriously.

Could it be the compounds my hands were in daily that led to this disease?

I don't know and probably never will.

Even if I found the answer, would it make this disease leave my body?

Nope, so I have to concentrate on things that help me, not the things that taunt me.

So, what am I gonna do – focus on that which I'll probably never find out, or contend with the battle at hand?

That's a no brainer.

I'M GOING TO TRY TO EXPLAIN THE PIECING TOGETHER of clues to my ultimate diagnosis.

I've been significantly affected by heat, certainly in my military years. It didn't help that I was at a southern base that was 13 feet below sea level. That meant I was basically working in a mechanical shop in stifling heat and humidity and doing so for long hours to boot. I remember my face would almost explode in a cartoon*esk* red orb of excessive heat exposure. I'd have to run to the bathroom, pour water on my face and leave a soaking wet paper towel on it even as I went back to work in an effort to alleviate the agony. There was no AC in this old shop and the work I did required much physical exertion and stamina, so I had that going against me too.

Let's run this down:

I'm not from these parts. I'm from the north and not used to this weather.

We're 13 feet below sea level (otherwise known as swamp city).

The heat is unbearably intolerable.

I'm swelling from the inescapable humidity.

The job requires much physical exertion and stamina which amps up my adrenaline and blood pressure.

Oh, let's not forget those uniforms... AND we often wore heavy-duty coveralls over them to avoid damage and staining from the bulky tooling, mechanical greases, and compounds.

Talk about being placed in a microwave!

SUBSEQUENTLY, I GOT DIAGNOSED WITH ROSACEA AND suffered from it the whole time I was stationed there. Once I got reassigned to another more northerly base, I never had that issue again. That'll give you an idea of the temperature my body was exposed to every spring, summer, and fall.

I'm mentioning this because I had an acute sensitivity to heat and humidity, and I thought it was due to relocating from the north to the south. That particular affliction stays with me to this day and is a huge indicator for people with MS – heat intolerance. That's only a slice of what was to come. Just when you think you've lived through the highest temperatures possible, I was proven wrong.

One of my assignments put me smack dab in a middle eastern desert. Let's talk colors for a moment. There's the average Joe white, then there's china doll or fluorescent white, and then there's me. I'm pretty much see-through and quite vascular. In fact, one of my nicknames in grammar school was "map" – I'll let you sort that one out on your own.

You know how when you cook bacon in a frying pan, it spits and sizzles? Well, that's me in an arid desert environment. My extremely blonde spiderweb-consistency thin hair facilitated the sun burning straight through to my scalp.

Awesome!

I'm pretty sure I used 100 power sunblock but would sweat it off instantly. Keep in mind you can't put sunblock on your scalp. I was tortured by the close, equator scorching from that fierce sun. It didn't take them very long to figure out there was no way I could survive on the dayshift.

So, off to nights I go and wow!

What a difference – *this* I can take. Still, it's the only time in my life that I've ever had coloring and I wasn't trying to do any of it. You just can't avoid it. Remember, I have not yet been diagnosed with MS, but the suffering commenced.

PER THE MILITARY WAY, I WAS REASSIGNED TO AN even more northerly base than my birth origins. To people with my sensitivity, that meant relief... FINALLY!

One summer, it was time for a break, so I took some leave to see my parents. They no longer lived up north and had moved down south. I didn't pay that any mind until I got there. It was literally like walking into a steamer, especially coming from the cool of the north. To give you a timestamp, this would've been in the very early 2000s. My heat intolerance not only came back instantly, but something else was added to the mix.

I remember snagging my leg on my mother's rosebush as a thorn caught my thigh. This was my first experience with what I call, 'the grid'. It's not just the specific ouch of a thorn in the thigh, it's the entire grid of nerves encompassing my upper leg being instantly and painfully electrified. If I poked my finger anywhere on my upper leg, the entire grid would spark in its shorted electrical wiring!

It was such an alien sensation to me.

Even the light swiping of my hand across the cutaneous level of my skin had the same painful, firing effect. I remember having a mystical look on my face like, what the f--- is that? It wasn't done though; it took on a creepy manifestation that actually stayed with me for around six months.

EVEN THOUGH MY LEG WORKED FINE, IT WAS MY FIRST time experiencing the numbness, and pins and needles sensation from my rump down. It would not go away no matter what over-the-counter Advil/Tylenol type pain reliever I tried. Fed-up, I just tolerated it for about three months and eventually relented to go see a doctor. He thought I may have pinched a nerve in my back and told me to do light duty for a while.

Sure...because that's *j u s t* how life works!

It took another three months to dissipate but, I just chucked it off as a fluke occurrence and pressed on. These episodes would occur a couple of times a year.

Fast forward to years in the future...

I was handed a copy of my medical records to bring to an appointment, so I thumbed through them. Had I not been handed a copy of my medical records, I never would have known that the Doctor wrote down that it was 'Paresthesia'. That's a word I would've remembered hearing, but he never said that to me.

The numbness and pins and needles feeling resurfaced several times a year and lasted for numerous months at a time. Because of what he had originally told me, I kept affiliating that sensation with the possibility that I just hurt my back again and it would fade away. As I said, it was a returning symptom during my insanely busy and intense work life. I didn't have time for this crap. It was in my way, so I kept on keeping on.

Just so you know, pins and needles and numbness are often quite prevalent in patients with MS. In fact, a lot of people remember 'Paresthesia' as being their first MS symptom. Patients often experience years of freakish physical anomalies and false guesses before the eventual proper protocol of testing leads to an MS diagnosis.

It's not the doctor's fault.

We're in these bodies ourselves and scratching our heads too. Thankfully, the diagnosing of this disease is so much more streamlined now. OK, so back to location, it's time for another assignment.

NOW, IN A JOB UTILIZING MY EXACT EXPERTISE, I'M chomping at the bit to begin my new work. The adrenaline and motivation have me invigorated and extremely pleased with both the new job and the fact that I am the best person to do *exactly* what I'm doing.

I'm a workaholic and it's not a chore, it's a love affair. However, something resurfaces, and I don't understand why it keeps happening. For so many years, decades really, I experienced severe molar and jaw pain. I wrote a story later in this book that explains the repeated diagnosis of trigeminal neuralgia which is the worst pain to experience.

Look it up.

It's the nerve that goes across your jaws and through to your teeth.

I'll give you an understanding of the massive intensity of this particular debilitating pain. It's so bad, even breathing hurts, talking hurts, and forget swearing. That's out. Any temperatures of hot or cold put me in the fetal position of pain. You don't even want to eat, let alone brush your teeth. In my case, I don't even want to move my mouth or make facial expressions of any kind because it's in my cheeks too. Believe me, I'm an expressive talker so this stopped me dead in my tracks. Do you know how hard it is to communicate when you have that much pain while in a new job?

Dear Lord, what is going on?

Trigeminal Neuralgia also follows several people who have MS (remember, it's a nerve). This disease attacks your own nerves, and it doesn't care what it targets in its relentless pursuit for damage. I will break this particular nightmare down in its entirety later on.

Let me explain my history here.

The military had previously performed jaw surgery on me, and my primary care doctor wondered if complications were manifesting from that. So, he sent me to an ear nose and throat (ENT) specialist. That doctor wants the backstory which I can barely tell him from the pain I'm in.

He then sends me off for an MRI.

SINCE I LOANED HIM MY MEDICAL RECORDS FOR HIS evaluation and it was almost a month of not hearing anything back, I called. Via phone, the receptionist tells me that the doctor can't speak to me – he's busy. So, a couple of days later with the same result, I stopped in. The receptionist again attests that the doctor is still too busy, but in her young, very flippant teenage-ish style voice, she says very matter-of-factly,

"Oh, he thinks you have MS".

What??

My lightning speed response was to say, 'He's on crack! I don't have MS! Give me my records', and to bolt out the door. What my brain processed was relative to muscular dystrophy which affects the muscles. I'm STRONG... a force to be reckoned with, physically (back then).

I get back to work and repeat the story to my co-workers. The receptionist's words have me very perplexed and insulted. What doctor lets his receptionist say words like that with no medical explanation?! My coworkers and I were all in agreement that this lady's nuts and the doctor's a butthole for not coming out and explaining this to me! Clearly, I had no clue what this disease actually was, so surfing I go.

What the hell is multiple sclerosis?

First of all, I was completely wrong in my assumption of what I *thought* she meant. I confused two diseases affecting the muscles versus the nerves.

Second of all, one of the most dangerous things I did was to surf for information. At that time (around 2008), it told me lies about people with MS having to stop working, driving, and being confined to a wheelchair in 2 years!

WRONG!

I worked for another 10 years after my diagnosis, almost 20 years after the first symptoms. Everybody's different and will experience different symptoms at different times with varying intensities. Please use reputable websites for your information, like the National Multiple Sclerosis Society (nationalmssociety.org), the MS cando-ms.org, or the MSworld.org sites, to name a few. Boy, do I wish I knew about those in the beginning of my MS journey.

So, back to the first time that receptionist said MS to me.

I was referred to a neurologist who conducted the physical evaluation and scheduled me for a spinal tap.

Holy freaking cow, Batman!

Spinal taps are no fun and quite weirdly painful... *but don't you move!* I remember when he took what felt like a javelin out of my spine. The sensation of it jammed into the vertebra and did not go away. Well, at least not for a couple of days. That's what I mean by weird. They also drew my blood at that time. Weeks later at a follow-up Neurology appointment, the MS diagnosis was unfortunately confirmed.

The MRI showed the icky lesions in my brain which is also indicative with this disease. The spinal tap lab results showed the tell-tale higher number of certain proteins. Don't ask me the details – I'm not a doctor. Google it or ask your doctor, better yet. To bring you back to where I was at...

I wasn't buying it.

NOPE, NOPE... THIS CAN'T BE RIGHT. I NEED A SECOND opinion.

After thorough research, I hard pursue a neurologist who specializes in MS. His bio was really impressive. As far as this disease is concerned, he turned out to be fate. His assessment of me physically for my functionality blew-my-mind! He was assessing many of the things that were oddities I had shrugged off as a fluke.

What a very impressive doctor and experience.

Unfortunately, he too confirmed the diagnosis.

So, that's the original ENT who, by the way, never told me his suspicion. He had his receptionist do that part. Plus, a neurologist, and a second opinion from an MS specializing neurologist – all confirmed the diagnosis of multiple sclerosis.

Note this: a thorough interview where they ask you relevant questions for matters indicative of this disease, a physical movement including motor skills examination, an MRI with contrasting fluid so the suspect lesions can glow, a spinal tap, and bloodwork.

That's the necessary mixture for a proper MS diagnosis.

I'm laying this out right now because I've heard horror stories of a "*Doctor*" who immersed his patients in a hot sauna to see if they were affected by the heat?! That's how this clown would diagnose MS! I find that to be a crime because it causes that person unnecessary, dangerous and stressful, panicked exposure to heat, let alone literally causing nerve damage!

OK, OK, back to legit stuff.

One of the questions asked to MS patients is about numbness, and pins and needles (Paresthesia). Then, it was almost 8 years since I had experienced that first episode of that particular symptom. It's unfortunately all too common to have a very wide gap of years between the first symptoms and the ultimate diagnosis of MS. That time in purgatory of not knowing what's going on with your body adds to the stress of the unknown. Remember, and I'm saying this in hindsight...

Stress is the enemy.

I'M NOT A DOCTOR AND I DON'T PLAY ONE ON TV, BUT I am living in the stink of this disease.

Here's my definition:

Multiple Sclerosis is where your central nervous system is under attack by your own immune system. Your body thinks it's an alien and the nerves don't belong there. Specifically, it's where the Myelin sheath (coating) around the nerves get attacked. That's called the demyelination of the central nervous system.

For a comparison, remember the candy called Good & Plenty that had the black licorice inside and the candy coating (pink and white) on the outside? If you pinched a piece of that candy, it would create cracks in the sugar-coating surface (sheathing) and expose the licorice (nerve). The nerve's exposure is what happens due to the Myelin sheath around it being attacked and damaged, creating the opportunity for the neurological damage of MS. Wherever that nerve is in your body translates to (Head, hands, brain, bladder, legs, eyes... Etc.), causes the neurological oddities of MS.

Multiple Sclerosis is a progressive disease and as of today, there is no cure. The way MS damages your nerves can also be exacerbated by 1000 different things. For instance, stress, body swelling... i.e., heat or humidity exposure, infections, lack of sleep or an improper diet, to name a few. Your own behavior can exacerbate your condition and worsen it. Anxiety, for example, also likes to tag along with this disease. This part of the MS experience was a very tough learning curve for me as the hits come faster than you can sort out resolutions, especially when you have not yet been diagnosed.

IT'S TANTAMOUNT TO TRYING TO TAKE A BREATH WITH your face upwards in a waterfall. Think back and recall all those times I said I was working under extreme heat and humidity, as well as intensity and stress – all negative players in this sickening tsunami.

MS likes to target specific categories in its damage, things like the eyes/vision, walking and gait problems, balance, speech, cognition, motor skills, dexterity, bladder and bowel disfunction (neurogenic), paresthesia, the dreaded MS "hug" as we MS'ers call it.

There's so many more and not everyone experiences the same symptoms. The disease is often referred to as the 'snowflake effect' in that you never know when and where a snowflake will hit your body. All of these things and many more came to pass in my life, but this story is to show you the beginning.

There was a six or seven-year span between my first symptoms and the first proper diagnosis. I've been suffering from the ridiculousness of this disease for just under 20 years. None of us have the same experiences because none of us are the same person. We have different loads of responsibilities and stressors, as well as different eating patterns and sleeping patterns. There's no 1-shot here – this is a gaggle f---ing disease and I'm down for the fight.

I have no choice.

Put any opposition in front of me, and good luck – the battle is on!

It's me and MS in the cage and I'm not gonna lose.

I'M NOT TELLING YOU TO FIGHT.

I'm letting you know there's another option than to lay down and take it. I am alive right now and will be until the day I find myself at the feet of my gracious creator. I'm not a calm person, but I can find pockets of peace and enjoy them. My MO is more combative to evil or wrong, and if I could help it, I would, but I can't.

Having said that, MS has quite the adversary in me. I'm absolutely convinced a cure for this disease will be found in my lifetime as they are making significant strides every day. I had to jot down the very beginnings of my MS experience. The following chapters will be imbedded in the nightmare of the pepper spraying of the disease's bombardment of damage on me. I desperately want to get off this ride, but apparently, I'm belted in this twister round-up ride of cruelty. The hits keep coming as the next chapters will depict.

Not to worry though, there are peaceful pockets... forced, beautiful moments. It's not all gloom and doom, and I wrote this book basically to let people know that you're not the only one. We're out here experiencing the same things. It doesn't even matter if you have MS or any other disease for that matter. There is a way to function and succeed against the obstacles placed in front of you. I am living proof of that very thing.

So, buckle your seatbelt, because we're going for a ride!

SANDY O.

2

MARY JO WAS MY FRIEND – SHE IS YOUR NEIGHBOR

DEC. 28

So, I'm lazy today and lounging on my couch, scrolling through estate sale listings.

It's Saturday.

There's several going on when I see what catapults me off the couch in shock – It's Mary Jo's address!!!???

I scream, "I KNOW HER!"

Dear God, did she die?

Was she put in a home?

Guilt and panic are the instant sensations of the day, the week, the month, and the lesson will be with me forever.

I THREW YESTERDAY'S CLOTHES ON AS FAST AS I COULD and darted over to her house. I am confronted with a sea of people with my usual *'make a penny scream'* mentality of estate sale'ing.

I have to find out what happened to her?

They're taking names for procession of entry. I go up to the security guard on the front porch to see what he can tell me – he has no details. I'm there with my out-of-town brother who can't make heads or tails of my reaction, but I am quite beside myself. I am Mary Jo's friend!

You see, Mary Jo lived close by and is the sweetest woman you'll ever meet. I knew she was up there in age, but she was positively full of life and joy.

In my insanely busy work existence, I saw her in transit from work and always stopped to catch up if I saw her in her driveway. She would talk about the art class she taught and how she loved it. She invited me to attend and browse the class. You see, I adore art – we had that in common. I was an artist in my younger years, so she and I enjoyed that common thread. I want you to remember what I'm writing here as it relates to an 'F' on my personal report card later.

I've been in Mary Jo's house several times but just to check in on her, pass the time, and see if she needed anything. I first met her during early 2008's massive ice storm. She was one of so many elderly people in my neighborhood living alone and I coordinated the movement of them to their in-the-neighborhood friends who had power. Those who wouldn't leave their non-powered houses, I brought food and coffee to. Since I left my name, address, and phone number with them all so they could tell their families who was working with them, Mary Jo was one of several who also took my invitation to use my storm shelter during inclement tornado weather.

Ironically, it turns out she had her own storm shelter all along. That goes to show people just want to have a conversation and enjoy the company of a neighbor.

She's been to my house several times where I showed her my

artwork and the pieces I collected. She clearly loved it too and once again explained she taught art at the local community college, inviting me to her class. I said I'd go, but it is dependent on my work demands. I never made it to that tour, but boy did I work myself into poor health.

In hindsight, not taking her up on touring that class is a huge lifetime regret for me. It was such a small thing I could've done to be a vessel to let her show me her passion.

Fast forward to that estate sale – my name is finally called.

THE HOUSE IS FULL, AND I DIDN'T CATCH WHAT I SAW until the end of round one – her house is the same as when I visited her – everything is still there! It felt like I was invading her privacy and it made me feel very uncomfortable and sad. I avoided the crowd and banked right to the 1st door on the right.

I am instantly floored!

I've never explored her house. I've just sat with her in her living room and passed the time. The room I'm in now is her art room – her paintings, her drawings, her instructional and inspirational books...

WOW!

More importantly, it's the beginnings of her masterpieces.

I AM IMMEDIATELY SURROUNDED WITH HER TALENTED works, her broad skill sets, and certainly, the knowledge that I have failed to learn more about her. I am asking the art room tenet (a male estate sale worker), if he knew if she passed away or got moved to a retirement home. He, too, had no info.

It was not the first thing I did in that room.

To the right, on the floor, is a stack of her art. I dove down to the most beautiful charcoal drawing. Its light shown down on a city street, glaring to a man's little vendor's cart. The cart's white and contrasting red striped umbrella is the point of the sun's accent in the hazy-day drab of a city street. It's in my hands and I can't believe the perfection I'm looking at! I went back to the house to get the charcoal she presumably used to draw it.

I am learning more about her looking at her work.

I SET THAT PICTURE ASIDE ON THE SOLD TABLE SO I can continue my quest to find out more about what happened to her. My brother guarded that table as he, too, saw the extraordinary beauty in the artist's rendering. In fact, he stopped someone from stealing that picture – a common problem with estate sales and why security is needed at them. The security guard stopped a few "accidental" lifting of things off the sold table. I found out later that the staff were equally taken aback by her artwork and acquired her pieces too.

This is a testament to her unsung talents.

My discussions with several of the people at the sale who knew her were so sad.

Mary Jo did pass away.

I was, and am, so crushed. Even more startling was what I found out in my internet searching that night – she passed away a year and a half ago!

How could I not know that?

It was a time stamp for me and a gauge of how long I'd not been well. I then realized that I changed my phone number around the same time as her passing.

She couldn't have had my new number.

HOW MUCH LONELINESS AND AILING MUST SHE HAVE been going through and without being able to call on me?

This is the 'F' failing grade I was referring to above.

All of us are drops that make up the bucket of water – we're each ingredients to a life experienced.

I knew <u>Mary Jo</u> had a son but found out she actually had two!

Again, my failing for not knowing more about her and giving her my time.

I couldn't wrap my head around how he could sell his mother's art.

It was beyond me.

I eventually made it upstairs and absolutely lost it – full-on uncontrollable tears. There was a beautiful, joyous picture of her holding her son as an infant. I was affected deeply that it would even be for sale and didn't understand how these things, her precious things, could be sold? I proceeded to her bedroom and felt honored to see what she saw when she went to bed. There was a stunning portrait of a lady in a draped towel, presumably fresh from a bath, and a landscape painting that took my breath away – it hung above her headboard.

I perceived her pride in these paintings, which explained their placement to be enjoyed by their creator. I had to have that which she saw every night. At some point, I found out there was some conflict in the family. It turns out one brother bought the other brother out and sold everything. I then found another similar picture of her holding the second son. I bought that one too.

My mission had completely changed.

I KNEW GIVING MARY JO HER DAY IN THE SUN WAS absolutely paramount.

Just because you're unpublished and not in the limelight doesn't mean you don't deserve to be recognized for your talents and brought into the light to be appreciated. There were numerous people moved by her work and they were buying her art.

I preserved as much of her art as I could afford, to be able to show the spectrum of her work. I gathered some family pictures and a pictorial collage of her for a snapshot of her legacy. Going back five times, I gathered a bouquet of things to respect the artist:

Numerous pieces of her artwork demonstrating her varied capable skills (oil paintings, charcoal works, portraits...etc.).

I bought her wooden suitcase she used as an easel for her work, her charcoal, a couple of books I thought she clearly referred to in her landscape paintings (which were done to perfection), a famous artist book, her wooden "Mary" engraved jewelry box, a wooden bowl with age of use...etc.

The family pictures I gathered were intentional as well. I wanted to be able to facilitate any healing in the family and begin a new joy of their mother. I, too, am the recipient of a healing of my family from the kind, insightful words of a good Christian man. Here I am with my brother whom I have a healed relationship with, at this estate sale, and I knew God brought me here.

I'm certain now.

I LEFT MY NAME WITH THE ESTATE SALE PEOPLE asking them to have the son call me.

He did not.

I called back to remind them I would work with the community college to show her art and allow her actual students that were inspired by her to obtain her works at no cost benefit to me. There are pieces I will keep as a lover of art and of her work. It's her beautiful pieces of art I'm trying to preserve for the students as well as family items recoverable through their healing. I have learned more of who she was during this experience than I knew of her alive. That's a lesson for me and hopefully of use to the readers.

That neighbor next door or down the street...

Perhaps you never see them, or they never open their blinds, or the one you wave to as you drive by in your busy day – they're a complete person and you might hold their bucket's missing drop of water.

They're often in need of company, to just talk, or show who they are or were. They're a drop in your bucket and make us complete too. I can tell you this – everything Mary Jo drew is alive!

YOU CAN SMELL THE SALTY WATER, HEAR THE windblown rustle of the leaves, engage with the eyes of her portraits, hear the streams as they pass in her landscapes, experience the cold dreariness of a sailor's gloomy dock, and relish the abstract beauty of her charcoal depictions. Her work is so alive and must be seen and appreciated. I am now her biggest fan and only wish I could've shown her the attention she and her artwork deserve.

Never shade a blooming, sun-thirsty flower.

Mary Jo was a woman of small stature, hair entwined in a bun. She was always smiling, always had kind words, and was an example for people, like me, who still need to pick up those traits. I recall seeing her little car go to and fro and remember her being more active than I was.

My world was work, work, work, work, and mom assignments sprinkled with the joy of art.

She is definitely one to use as an example. I found out from her obituary that she was very well educated. She earned a BS in zoology, one course away from earning a Master's in chemistry. <u>Mary Jo</u> was married for 40 years and had several jobs of service including helping her husband's dental practice and being a pediatric technician. She was active in her church and a wonderful person to converse with and know. I miss her very much and will brag about her forever.

You may have noticed that I am not using her last name – that's intentional. The release of that is up to her family. You may also have noticed I am underlining her name – that too is intentional to show respect for both her name and how she signed her drawings.

I would love to see all her works as many left her house before I could see them. I hope to help reveal her hidden talents and beautiful artwork.

Please take the meaning from my drop in the bucket neighborly true story. This could be happening to any one of us. Nobody should die alone… to be forgotten. Isolation can run tandem with MS. Reaching out to people who are going through some significant things is very needed.

We're human after all.

MS can absolutely make you feel like you're the only one experiencing these things, but you're not. It's very important to reach out to the MS community by way of sites like MS world, or the national multiple sclerosis society, and the MS Can-Do organization, for example. All three of those have been extremely instrumental in my life both in understanding this disease and in fellowship with people who are experiencing the same baffling symptoms.

Again, MS sucks.

Let's not let people squander away in isolation.

. . .

SANDY O.

MARY JO WAS MY NEIGHBOR. SHE WAS AN EXCEPTIONAL
artist and human being, and I miss her. Let's please be
neighbors and fill those empty buckets.

SANDY O.

3

OH YEAH? TAKE THAT!!!!

MAR. 5

THE DREADED JAR.

Ughhh!

OPEN!!!!

Friggin' OPEN!!!

Stupid hands!

Enter stage right: rubber gripper pads. Put those rubber grip pads on top of a jar and voila. I will have my sweet pickles. Denial of function is NOT going down without a fight. You got the wrong one, MS!

Take THAT!

OK, HERE GOES.

I can't flip an egg with a spatula anymore. So, I spray Pam on the bottom of the pan as well as the top then flip them whole, in the pan (over the sink, of course). I can't peel, slice, or shred hash brown potatoes anymore.

So what!

Instead, I cut them into little cubes. They look different, but it tastes great, and I can do it. Potatoes I shall have (my favorite food). Maintaining a hold of my heavy straight up-and-down drinking glasses escapes me these days, so I replaced my frustrating glasses with a $10 estate sale find.

Eight lightweight crystal stem wine glasses.

Those don't slip out of my hands because they increasingly bow outward as well as having a stem to grab onto for added control. Those glasses helped me out so much, but my clumsiness would cause them to easily break, so I've since upgraded them to a meatier, large-stemmed wine glass for my drinks. I don't drink alcohol but, boy oh boy, does it sure hold lots of water and is so much easier for me to handle.

So... voila.

Take THAT!

THIS ONE WAS VERY TOUGH FOR ME.

I'm at lunch with a co-worker talking about the barrage of symptoms I'd been increasingly affected with, when I couldn't maintain hold of the restaurant's utensils. They were too heavy and bulky, and by now, I'm covered in food. I was completely defeated, scared, embarrassed, and crying like a baby. I never went back to work again.

It was my last day.

The weight of the cornucopia of symptoms I was dealing with really *put the screws on me* and I needed help dealing with all this. So, I saw a psychiatrist to help me deal with the barrage of physical losses I was experiencing and in such a rapid progression. She was of tremendous help to me. It helped me think and process things differently. I'm now applying the same techniques I used in my technical career towards my MS symptoms.

. . .

IF FORKS CAN TAKE ME OUT OF COMMISSION, I NEEDED to bring myself back in. I found a $5 set of plastic lightweight round-handled silverware at an estate sale.

Problem solved!

The same is true for holding a round handled cup for my green tea. Those roll down in my looped fingers. I quickly ditched those for square handled cups. None of my cups match, but they all work, and they all hold my tea so...

Take THAT!

HERE ARE MORE CASES-IN-POINT:

My balance can be thrown off when I bend down to pick things up. So, I bought several extended grabber devices (I have one in most rooms) at a buck a piece.

Yes, estate sales... and they're awesome.

Using my toothbrush was next to impossible. I couldn't maintain the finite grip or twist of it. Thanks to my occupational therapist, I now have these foam one-inch grips to cut to size. I stick my toothbrush in it and I'm back to center. She hooked me up with all kinds of assistive devices to help me pour, button, arrange my pills...etc. She was awesome and very knowledgeable. When things are everyday needs and those functions fail, I scream and cry, but only for a few minutes. I'm not interested in wallowing in my own pity party for long. Revenge on behalf of my body is what's required here. I was never the passive type and I'm not going to start that with MS.

SO, I HAD TO GO BACK TO WORK FOR MYSELF TO regain my functions. If you're not used to saying no to something, say it now. I fight to maintain everything, albeit in a different way. Who cares how you do it so long as you're trying?

Listen, I'm not delusional. I've experienced things that are changed forever. I get aggravated and loud, and then I press the heck on. I lost my ability to be outside in the heat or humidity, so I was prescribed a cool vest. It's a way of having a solution to an outside event I can't miss.

I will make that annual Art Show!

Solutions are the name of the game and I seek them out. Even asking your doctor, your therapists, or your support groups is seeking a solution.

Stay empowered and ask!

I HAVE PLENTY OF UNMENTIONABLE THINGS I removed from this story in an effort to maintain my dignity. We all do or will deal with plenty of unmentionables. Continuing, I used to have to use a shower chair due to falling all the time. Your doctors will help you medically to stop the exacerbations and relapses. Your therapists will walk you through the recoveries, but YOU must be gainfully employed in the recovery of your own body.

That doesn't mean you have to physically do everything yourself – it's ok to ask for help when you need it. It's important to check yourself regularly to make sure you still need the assistive devices you're using.

Test it.

Test your work's progress.

If you don't need it, get it out of your sight! If you need it, install it and use it. It's not a crime to be impaired. We've been the unwelcoming recipients of what this disease imposes on us. So, with assistance close by, I showered without the shower chair and found the hard work I was doing paid off. I'm still standing up in the shower for the last two years. What a pleasure, and I count those.

Are you?

It's small to everyone who stands during a shower. It's

HUGE to anyone who *has* to sit down. Where you are today may not be where you are tomorrow...remember that.

EVERYTHING'S DIFFERENT NOW.

I have to be in my very small square shower.

I have to touch the walls when my eyes are closed.

I had to change from squeeze bottles to trigger pump style ones.

It's safer for me to towel off in the seated position rather than standing...so that's what I do. I insist on working on my progress.

Is every day the same?

Absolutely not, but I'm doing it.

Am I stubborn?

All signs point to yes.

Determined?

You Betcha!

I'm unapologetic about that.

HERE ARE MORE FRUSTRATIONS THAT I DEAL WITH:

The MS medicine I was on made my hair fall out and get very thin. Add in the insane itching of Facial Myokymia and all bets are off.

I'm pissed!

Throw in the fact that I couldn't put my hair up anymore due to finite dexterity issues.

FINNNNNNE!

This is WAR!

I asked my neurologist about this and got fantastic advice. I added BIOTIN to my daily supplements for my hair. For me, it worked. My hair is much healthier. To offset the itching issues, I had my long hair cut short. That was so empowering and immediately removed the stress my hair had caused me for years. Removing stress is an essential ingredient for my health. You know, it's an integral part of a woman... her hair.

But guess what...

I won this fight, MS didn't.

This is how my type-A self-deals with the war being played against my body. I know there's plenty coming my way in the progression of this disease, but I owe it to myself to retain as much as I can.

WHEN IT'S APRIL IN TORNADO ALLEY, I CLEAN OUT MY tornado shelter. I get the spiders out and replenish the water and snacks. Come May, the sirens will blow, and I'll be sitting in the safety of my storm shelter.

Plan your functional repairs that way.

I give it all I've got in the counterattack. Like, in cards, you need to know when to fold them. Some things you just can't do, maybe never again.

You'll know the difference.

I stopped driving when I couldn't feel my feet. Once removed from my work stresses and with the assistance of my Neurologist and physical therapist, my situation started turning that right around. The feelings in my feet came back and I've been driving for well over two years now. However, I will stop immediately if I can't feel my feet again.

This is what I've learned.

If you're always laying on the couch, you'll have a PhD in laying on the couch. Get up, if you can, and move a little. Get up two days later and move a little more. Execute the counterattack on what this disease is trying to take from you. Enact a plan towards recovery with your medical staff's involvement /approval.

· · ·

SOME OTHER PROGRESS EXAMPLES FOR ME ARE:

I used to be unable to do the heel-to-toe walk for my doctor. I lost that, I assume, in the lesions and black holes in my brain. My physical therapist let me know – the average person uses a small percentage of their brain for daily functions.

So, I read an article called, "Do People Use Only 10% of their Brains?" It was on "ScientificAmerican.com" and written by Robynne Boyd on Feb 7, 2008. The article had a line in it that resonated with me. It said something like, "after injury or even after partial brain removal, the brain has a way of compensating and making sure that's what's left takes over the activity."

How cool is that?

My physical therapist said, through repetition, rewire that heel-to-toe function to another part of your brain. She said to stop using my arms on the walls to stop my imbalance. Instead, pop my leg out for the correction.

Guess what... it worked!

Each time it takes me 2 or 3 attempts, but then I can do heel-to-toe. Even typing this story is an exercise in fighting to regain what I lost in finite dexterity. Now, this is my personal experience.

Work is required if you want results.

TWO YEARS AGO, MY TYPING WAS FRAUGHT WITH TYPOS every other letter and I raged in frustration. My handwriting was completely unreadable. When I had the idea of this story, I got out a paper tablet, a pen, and hand wrote the notes for this. My intentional hand uses paid off.

I could read all my notes!

Practice = rewiring.

Be Stubborn!

MS is trying to determine who you are. You have to be more stubborn than it is. This is war! Gear up, eat well, move more, practice with repetition, talk with your medical personnel, and use (in your own way) the advice of people who've been there and acquired their own successes.

Take command of your own body and insist on your role in your body's recovery.

LET'S BE HONEST, I'M NOT IMMUNE TO THE FULL LOSS of a function.

We're all going to have to deal with that. It is a progressive disease... for now. I have hope and my faith. However, clean out your storm shelters in April for the May tornado sirens...in Tornado Alley.

It's a guarantee.

So is MS and the losses you must take charge of, either by physical actions, and/or by adjusting your attitude.

I've adopted something that works for me. I owe it to myself to try and try again.

When I couldn't work the posts of an earring, I switched to the slide-in style.

Can't perform a screenshot on your iPhone anymore? Here's your solution: Go to your iPhone's settings icon, General, Accessibility, Assistive Touch, enable it and voila! You'll have everything as a 1-touch function! BTW, other smart phones have that function too. So, go take that screenshot or the many other options. OBTW, get a 'POPSOCKET' or similar device to affix to your phone to assist in holding it.

When I couldn't press the spritz top of a perfume bottle, I poured it into a squeeze nozzle type bottle I found at the local drug store.

I couldn't work the little round twist-on of a lamp, so I bought a $10 touch lamp – best purchase I've made MS-wise.

Light I shall have!

. . .

HERE WAS MY BIGGEST HURDLE.

I had an intense career I loved for 30 years. I ate it up. It was such a pure sense of accomplishment. Enter vertigo, a neurogenic bladder, double vision, esotropia, pins and needles, canes, walkers, toilet seat handles...and the list goes on.

It changed everything.

I thought what I experienced all those years was the good kind of stress, you know, the kind I was wired for. I had to face the hard facts that MS changed how my body processed stress.

I had to cry UNCLE!

I've been disability retired for a few years now. Had I not done that, I wouldn't have been able to tell you how much better off I am, having removed myself from the stress. By paying attention to my own body's recovery, I have been able to draft/handwrite and type this story.

Night to Day/Dark to Light/Rage to Peace (I'm still working on that one).

I'm a work in progress and always will be. Once you accept that and forgive yourself for your own frustrations, you can move on and engage in life again.

SO, GET OUT THERE AND FIND OR START YOUR MS support group – it's priceless. We're all in this together and I've been rescued from my bad days by my MS group. I think I've helped others cheer up too. This is certain – we all look forward to the next meeting, we all have fun, and love each other's company.

Granted, COVID-19 changed everything to Internet meetings, but it's still a connection. Get out there and engage in life again – no isolation allowed (unless that's your nature). I know we all have different issues, different attitudes, and varying diagnoses, as well as different levels of responsibilities and stressors. I do not want to preach for anyone to use this

SANDY O.

story as a recipe but use it for inspiration to devise your own plan.

WE'RE HERE AND WE COUNT. SO, TO END WHERE I started, **Oh Yeah? TAKE THAT!!!!**

SANDY O.

RRMS BEGRUDGED RECIPIENT

TYPE A – SO THERE!

4

SAVOR THE AHHS

MAR. 9

I WENT THROUGH QUITE a bit with this disease, but I am currently stabilized. It took a lot of work. In my recovery, something quite profound happened. It took over a year to manifest, but I can hear the birds now.

I HAVE NO LIMITING HEARING ISSUES, BUT WHAT MY previous stressful life caused was a cloaking of all things good. Things I forgot – I needed serene sounds that I desperately missed. I had to get to a point of peace and relaxation to hear the birds again. They wake me up through my cracked bedroom window. There's nothing more pleasurable than a cool breeze coming through and being awakened by singing birds announcing the new morning. So, I consciously started collecting and savoring the Ahhhs.

THIS ONE LITTLE ACT WAS RESPONSIBLE FOR augmenting my peace. I love birds and always have. I feed them now and enjoy watching them come in to eat. They dance and sing for their potential mates. Their babies learn to feed here now, and they all compete with the squirrels in fighting for that last sunflower seed. I can settle in and enjoy the birds now. Cool morning air is offset by layers of blankets up to my neck. I'm breathing in that cool air. It doesn't get any better. I enjoy so much now, so many simple things.

I STARTED ALLOWING ALL THINGS GOOD TO ABSORB into my skin, to be enveloped by my eyes, ears, and nose. I count them now and as a result, all my positive senses are alive. I remember one short trip in the car and how beautiful the sky was – and I am driving. It's one thing to drive, but it's another to acknowledge that you have the ability to drive today.

I'm counting my blessings.

TODAY, I RODE A TRIKE-BIKE FOR THE FIRST TIME ever.

Freedom with no worries of falling.

The excitement of meeting up with my support group made all this a reality. The fellowship and happiness of all of us is contagious. There's holding a baby, and then there's a mother pulling her baby close where she's absorbing the connection of the love with her child. That's what I learned to do with everything I see, hear, smell, or feel that affects me positively. I'm intentionally extending the experiences – giving them a longer shelf-life, if you will. I recall those for extended pleasure and peace.

I EVEN SLOW THE DESCENT INTO MY BED EVERY NIGHT. My left knee sinks into the pillow top and my right leg dangles for just a sweet second before it completely lands on the bed.

It's so relaxing and I look forward to that very simple descent every single night.

Sinking into the fluffiness of the mattress.

All pins and needles dissipate from the comfort of that descent. It's the little things you can recall at a whim to relive its joy.

I USED TO GO TO A FLEA MARKET EVERY ONCE IN A while, and it's a beautiful mixture of people and their genuine interactions. It brings me great joy as I see a teenage Caucasian male sitting next to an approximately 80 to 90-year-old African American male, and they're just chewing the fat and talking about whatever they're talking about.

They're enjoying each other's company.

Despite the overwhelming sell of the news, this warms my soul. It reminds me of how I grew up in the mass diversity of the big city. I recall this memory often for my own joy. Everything pursued is possible and I pursue sightings of beautiful interactions.

THE PATIO DOOR IS OPEN AND IT'S EARLY MARCH. THE cool, almost cold air rolls in and I need to breathe it. I suspect there's quite a lot of us that need to do that. When I'm overheated, I step out barefoot onto my patio's cold cement floor. It's an instant body air conditioner and I love it. Summer will be here soon, and I'll be encased in my air-conditioned house. So, for now, I will steal every cool moment I can. My first sip of my warm green tea in the now cool living room with that back door being open is everything. I'm not thinking of any of the negatives, only the beauty of the cold.

. . .

SANDY O.

I WANT YOU TO NOTICE THAT I DID NOT CONCENTRATE on all the entails of this disease. I am not even giving it a voice. All my efforts go to the intentional thought of the simple, free and easy things that I've been given to enjoy. I do not have MS during these moments. I have cooler air, I have singing birds, and I have great rest.

The last words I want to say is, "I HAVE."

SANDY O.

AHHHHHH...

5

A CURE FOR COUCH-I-TUS
APR. 2

LET ME OUT!

I want water.

Let me in!

Rub my back, FEED ME, chase me, SQUIRREL!

Yep, you got my drift. Go, get you a puppy!

IF LAYING ON THE COUCH IS YOUR ISSUE, YOU'RE hurting yourself. Lack of movement equals muscle atrophy and the worsening of your MS symptoms. No, I'm not a doctor but I play one on TV... joke, joke. If you have capabilities beyond laying on the couch, the best thing you can do for our ridiculous condition (MS), is to go rescue a puppy.

I RETIRED AND FOUND MYSELF ON THE COUCH WAYYYY more than I ever thought I would be. My goodness are puppies ever a pain in the butt, but boy oh boy, my legs are so much stronger now. I just wanted to lay there... just me and the remote (back when I had cable). Puppies refuse to let you have your sedentary ways.

I HAD AN OLDER DOG – 17 IN HUMAN YEARS, 119 IN canine years. She's more the speed I'm equipped for these days... or so I thought. In walks my daughter with a nine-month-old miniature beagle.

You've gotta be kidding me!

Good luck trying to ignore a whining little puppy who wants what she wants when she wants it. Last time I experienced this was when my daughter was an infant over 20 years ago. Now I deal with *her* daughter who happens to be a miniature beagle.

AT THAT TIME, MY DAUGHTER WAS IN COLLEGE. SHE would pop in and out between classes to get her laundry that I'd washed and folded for her. She lived here, ate here, showered here, but she was a daughter who was back-and-forth between college, job hunting, work, friends, and whatever the social life someone in their early 20s had.

So, who was taking care of the dogs?

Mwah!

OH, DID I MENTION THAT THE OLDER DOG I HAVE IS also hers?

However, since I'm the one that takes care of her and trained her, I'm the one she listens to. I also had to train the rambunctious little beagle NOT to do the bad stuff on the carpet, to stop chewing all the squishy things, to get off-my-couch (I lost that battle), and to not bite my fingers when offered lunch meat... Etc.

OBTW, none of the above is done in the sitting position on the couch.

KEEP IN MIND THAT THE PUPPY HAS TRAINED ME TOO. This dog is obsessed to-the-nines with the laser pen! My daughter got her hooked on that. I can't even walk next to the cabinet where it's stored without her body posturing in the stalking/freezing position.

Get it! Get it! Get it!

Schnitzskies, if I don't respond to her panicked whines and pleas, I'll never get to hear the antiques roadshow and how much that item is worth!

So, getting up I must do.

THERE ARE PERKS TO THE PUPPY TOO. SHE HAD removed years of age from my older lab. Our tug-of-war play with the now mutilated string braided rope has me constantly moving and tickles me pink. I suggested naming the dog Twister.

I lost.

She spins, runs, jumps, and does her laps around the coffee table as she wants to be chased – not that I can run. But I can at least make her think I'm chasing her. More importantly, I'm up and NOT on the couch. She has me moving all the time. Oh, by the way, I am also 'watching' one of my daughter's friends' dogs and have been for over a year. Sadly, I lost my wonderful 17-year-old dog, and eventually adopted a giant from the local pound. Just when I thought the beagle was crazy for the laser...

The giant (Anatolian shepherd mixed with greyhound?) surpasses her by leaps and bounds. And when I say leaps, I mean gigantic room covering leaps!

. . .

THE BIGGEST, MOST SURPRISING PERK OF THE PUPPY was the two dogs were connected at the hip, so-to-speak. Well, more like hip to knee. Just watching them snuggle up together was so adorable. Now she does that to the other two 4-leggers in the house. I even get up to cover them with a blanket and tuck them in. The sight of them and how connected they are to each other calms me.

So, there's another plus for getting a puppy.

We all need as much good Mojo as we can get. Good calming warm fuzzy feelings – food for the soul. I would even suggest, if you don't have any dogs, go to your local pet rescue and get a puppy AND a mature dog. You will see the same transformation I am trying to convince you of right now. They make you move more. You'll feel obligated to take care of them which will require you to tend to their needs.

THE MORE YOU LAY ON THE COUCH, THE MORE sedentary you become and the more atrophy you bring on yourself. Something happens mentally in that process that almost tells you, "I'm on the way out or on a downward spiral." The same way this puppy took years off my 17-year-old dog, is the same way she has removed so much of my sedentary existence, my feelings of defeat, and a settling for the demise of this disease. I was surprised to find the puppy reversed all of the above.

THE PHYSICAL STRENGTH I GAINED FROM TENDING TO this demanding little puppy turned me onto all sorts of other beneficial movements. During commercials, or just walking through the house, I stop and do deep knee bends for no reason except to prove to myself that I can do it and that it will benefit me strength-wise.

I'm not kidding, go get you a puppy! It will get you off the couch and it will train you that you can do far more than you think you can.

Yipe Yipe, SQUIRREL!!!

SANDY O.

6

MECHANICAL ME
JUNE 16

ALL I WANT IS ONE FRIGGIN' Puff's tissue.

I gently reach for one, you know, because *they're so delicate...* I'm DENIED!

I gently try again...no go!

Third strike you're out?

I don't think so. Forget you, MS! I grab a handful and WILL retrieve the one I want from the bundle.

I WIN!

When I have a bad day due to stress, lack of sleep, or being overheated, it seems the gentler I am in functioning throughout the house, the more apt I am to be hurt or fail in the attempted process.

IN MY ATTEMPTS TO DO THE MINUTIA OF THE DAY, like gently picking this up or gently opening that UPS nuclear-wrapped package with my medicine in it, it fails and denies me. When I have days like that, I benefit from 'man handling' everything. As a result, I am rewarded with that which I seek.

. . .

SIMILARLY, THERE ARE DAYS WHERE MY WALKING IS way off balance, but I have things I need to do around the house. One of the ways I counter my MS imperfections is by concentrating on only the thing I need to function. If I know I'm having a bad day and I have to do this or do that, I can't have a lackadaisical mentality about it. I think of myself as machinery, like a drill that needs to punch that hole. I'm pretty sure the drill is not thinking... *oh, it's hot in here – I need to turn the AC up* before I **mechanically twist my drill bit and cut into this metal.**

No, no, it's functioning deliberately and mechanically.

I HAVE TO MECHANICALLY VISUALIZE THE LEGS AND their movement, the feet and their placement, the forward trajectory and its intended destination and, by golly, it works. I'll warn you – it does tire you out when you concentrate so specifically about a simple function, but sometimes you have to do what you have to do to get-'er-dun! At those times, I am only thinking about the nerve endings dealing with the tasks. All my concentration goes to that one function, that one muscle group, and I treat it very mechanically both in visualizing the action and executing the task.

I've become an extremely capable robot executing the task of walking.

I TIRE EASILY BUT THE MACHINE DOESN'T IN THE TASK at hand until its completion. Somebody sent me a video once on YouTube that showed this young girl running a race around the track with other girls. She was in her 20s I think, and she was winning. Towards the end of the race, her coach stood at the finish line and she collapsed in his arms. She starts screaming, "Please help me, I'm hot...My legs, my legs...Where'd they go?"

The video was called "Catching Kayla" and shockingly, she has MS!

I DID NOT UNDERSTAND WHAT I WAS LOOKING AT.

It really took me a while to understand that she was not able to walk most times and that she did something to get her body to execute the task of running. What a remarkable video that began an internal look at everything I had succumbed to, everything I said, 'I can't do this, and I can't do that,' about. It was the seed to this growing plant that is teaching me that, I CAN. For me, being mechanically minded, I started turning the 'I cant's' into commands to my body of "You Will" ... like Kayla did on that track. This is the part I confessed to, that when I compartmentalize each task into its mechanical function, it can be tiring, much like Kayla collapsing at the finish line.

SO, YOU HAVE TO MAKE A CHOICE.

Are you more comfortable allowing each demise with MS or are you stubborn like I am and refuse to bow-out of the fight?

It's a personal decision.

I was deeply moved and intrigued by what Kayla did on that track but had denied many, many times in her life. Figuring that out became the legend to my map. They'll be times I'm too tired to figure this out, but it's on my to-do list if I'm denied a function.

FOR ME, COMPARTMENTALIZING EACH FUNCTION AND concentrating on the muscles, the intended movement, the brain's nerve schematic, and the task at hand works. I keep reading about advancement after advancement in the understanding of MS.

A couple of years ago, I learned through the National Multiple Sclerosis Society (NMSS) about how we're all in this together. The email connected to a video by a woman who had an extremely similar MS path to mine.

Her name was Palmer Kippola.

Like watching Kayla and how it became a legend to my can-do map, so too has this video impacted me, especially the bit about the gut. I always feel swollen in my gut. Ms. Kippola had seven steps in this video and there was something like, the 5R Gut something or other, that I intend to attempt.

Challenge accepted!

The alternative is, that I just always have a swollen gut and live with it. But that's not me. So, stay tuned and I will let you know how this attempt turns out for me – mechanical me.

SANDY O.

7
PAIN = STRESS = RAGE
JUNE 18

BURNED AGAIN... flat iron.

Can't do my hair.

Round 2 – curling iron... burned again!

Fingers not cooperating... That's 1.

Event to go to – nothing to wear.

Shirt's too short, bra's not lifting, a thousand flung clothes

Nothing compliments... That's 2.

Remain CALM!!!! Goose fabbbber!

Hot today – dangerous implications.

.... Stay CALM!!!!!

Recover... must recover – been waiting for this event for weeks.

Pressure's building.

Ok, ok. Exhale – round 3.

Putting shirt on.

Who's this in the mirror? Who is that fat, sagging chick?!!!

Confidence blown... That's 4!

Yesterday? FANTASTIC!

Saw ex co-workers – first time in years. Rejuvenated.

Denied happy day #2.

Body's revolting, but why?
Wait a minute – think this through.
Oh, right... little sleep last night.
That's right – FULL day yesterday.
Ex-work visit, getting gas, grocery shopping.
Depleted week's MS allotted energy.
Reality sets in – my fault.
Sacrificed for 'The Fantastic Day.'
You are forgiven. Forgive me... note to self.
Must minimize depleted energy's destructive intentions.
TV, it is – History Channel.
Damn, North Korea: Dark secrets!
Not entertaining evil today.
Ahhhhh, PBS – "NATURE"
Who can be mad at frogs?
No more rage allowed... disconnect.
Oooooohmm...
EH – not me.
MUST WRITE!

SANDY O.

8

COINCIDENTAL EPIPHANY
DEC. 12

FIRST OF ALL, I want to say a belated thank you to all who have served or are serving the citizens of our wonderful country.

IT'S VETERANS DAY.

I have such a wonderful feeling today with the cool air upon us.

Snow is in the forecast.

The arctic blast just made my symptoms relax and I feel very comfortable today, happy in fact. I spent yesterday preparing for the cold weather by covering the water spigots, putting the non-slip rugs down outside, changing the smoke detector batteries, replacing the air vent's filter... Etc.

So today, the plan is to relax.

REMEMBER WHEN YOU WERE IN SCHOOL AND YOU actually read the assignment and you actually did the required questionnaire?

Remember how good you felt when you got to school and knew you did your homework?

There was no fear.

That's how I feel today having done all the winter's to-do's (that I can do anyway). Now it's time to relax, drink too much coffee in the comfort of my own home and take naps just because. I ate lunch late so now it's time for a late dinner. I'm still feeling so happy and want to be amongst people. I never go out after dark as I don't feel it's safe for me should anything happen to the car. However, today is truly different – I am beaming with happiness.

What's a person to do?

I start to conjure the options.

I'VE NEVER DONE THIS BEFORE BUT I'M THINKING... it's Veterans Day (observed), and so many go to a national buffet on this day. I think it's mostly to meet and greet and, unfortunately, some need a free meal. It's dark outside and I go against my principles and head there. I'm in such a rare mood.

I DRIVE CLOSE BY AND SEE THE RESTAURANT'S parking lot is full. It makes me happy to know that people are getting the fellow companionship we all enjoy. However, it's too cold for me to stand outside in a line, so I press on, undeterred, knowing I will stop somewhere and enjoy my rare evening out. It's been way too many years since my symptoms stopped me from venturing out and dining alone. There will be no such speed bump tonight. Ah, I'll stop over there at Santa Fe's (a great steakhouse restaurant).

. . .

SANDY O.

NOT A LOT OF PEOPLE THERE TONIGHT – IN FACT, I'M the only one in this area so far. I get seated at the 'Single and Alone' section, but I'm fine with that. Megan is my waitress and she's perfectly pleasant and personable. After getting my drink order (root beer – a mood celebratory drink since I don't drink soda anymore), we began to talk about the menu and its options. Nothing quite suits but she's very accommodating and says they will make what I want. So, it's a salad – very similar to a Cobb salad. I am splurging and add a small order of their phenomenal fries. She puts the order in, and I realize, quite suddenly, where I'm at.

Megan came back and I began to explain.

THIS IS THE LAST PLACE I ATE ON MY LAST DAY OF work before I was ultimately disability retired. I wrote about this in my earlier story called, "Oh Yeah? Take THAT!!!!"

In that story, I explained how bad my symptoms were accumulating, and how I could not even pick up my silverware and wound up covered in my food.

This is the same place, a few years later!

Adding to the irony of the location is that I am one booth away from that symptomatic finality of my career. However, it is not a bad feeling, it's an epiphany of where I'm *not* at symptomatically. To be safe, though, I unwrap the napkin to inspect the silverware.

Whew!

They've changed their silverware to a less non-bulky style.

I am relieved.

SO, I'M EXPLAINING TO MEGAN, HAVING ALREADY TOLD her that I was disability retired, that I have not gone out to eat alone in a restaurant since that very day. The irony of the situation does not escape me. I think God is showing me the then-and-now of his daily blessings. I thought I was glowing before I left my house but now, I know I am beaming!

BY NOW, SEVERAL PEOPLE HAVE COME INTO THE restaurant and there's an older, single man seated behind me in the row I'm in. There's a couple by the windows, probably wondering why I took a picture of my food (which I never do). A group of millennials are to my left and I am in full view of them. I'm sure they're wondering why I'm smiling, all by myself. I am completely and totally present in front of this wonderful array of food provided the exact way I requested it (a side of guacamole, a side of fries, romaine lettuce please, a side of warm corn kernels and no bread, thank you for asking, Megan).

Yes!

I am able to eat with the silverware, able to pick up my root beer glass and drink out of it, able to crack open the peanuts, and certainly loving this long-missed experience. I'm present and perfectly aware of the exceptional joy of tonight.

THE BILL COMES AND MEGAN'S NO-DOUBT BEEN explaining my story to the manager, who states he's cut my bill in half. I definitely don't like to get anything I haven't paid for but the gesture's beautiful and very appreciated. I pay the bill in full but leave Megan more than double in the form of a tip. Her pleasantries added to my out-in-the-dark, long time coming dining experience. A simple series of gestures and circumstances have filled my bank of joy. I'm sure the bank's coffers will remain full for a long time and I won't forget the MS symptoms comparison lessons. I will revisit this experience periodically because it paid exponentially to my joy of life.

What an incredibly different story... the same restaurant, the same room, and two different circumstances that have been taught to me. It was such a beautiful evening, and I am still smiling, ear to ear, days later.

SO, MY LESSON FOR THE READING AUDIENCE IS THAT bad symptoms can absolutely be overcome with time and good things. So be brave and try to recognize all the tiny positives you've had.

Collectively, they add up to so much.

SANDY O.

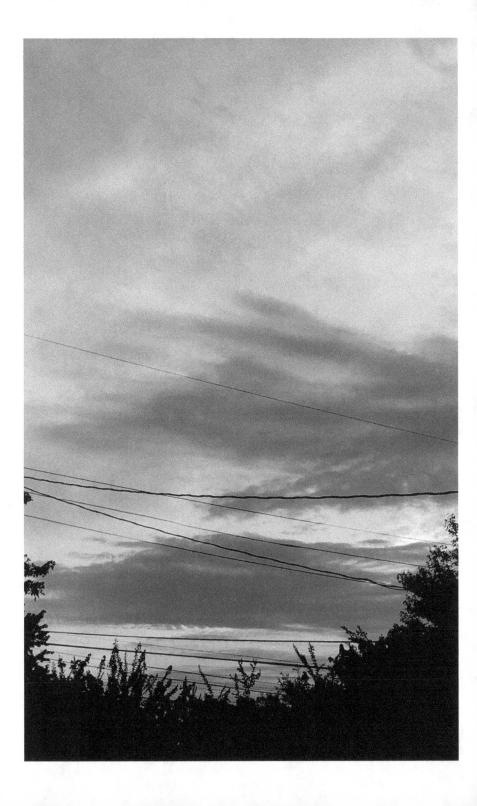

9

DO YOU SEE THE WIRES OR DO YOU SEE THE SKY?

DEC. 28

I USED to get up every morning between 3am and 6am to have oatmeal with the first round of my MS medicine. Believe me, I could easily complain that my retired butt is up too early in the morning but, for my health, I had to re-format my normal M.O. to stop concentrating on the negatives.

I now deliberately look for and appreciate the beautiful things.

WITH ME GETTING UP, THE DOGS ARE ALERTED TO OUR normal routine. It's time for them to do their business, which means food comes afterwards. So, after unlocking the back door –

<POOF!>

THERE'S THAT SKY!

WOW!

It demands my attention. The question is, can YOU see it?

DO YOU SEE THE INTRUSIVE WIRES OF LIFE, OR DO YOU see the delivery of that stunning sky?

It's a metaphor for the accruements of MS and how it's always laying wires to obstruct your view and block your joy in life. If you see the wires, you're like I was, and it's time for retraining. I suspect that, if you see the wires and *not* the sky, you may be also concentrating on the pins and needles, the pain, the imbalance, the vision issues, the malfunctioning limbs...etc., of MS. All these are not my symptoms, and they're certainly not all inclusive to the plethora of jinxes MS hits us with.

So, how can you *NOT* see the wires – metaphorically speaking?

There is a training plan to accomplish this. You learned to walk so, this too, is doable. Take that picture, for example.

I'VE ALWAYS SEEN THE GORGEOUSNESS OF NATURE BUT would contort myself to get that view to eliminate the ugly of industry in my shot. However, I've recently begun to overlook the so-called ugly markings of industry's footprints in lieu of the unquestionable beauty of nature. After all, my iPhone took that picture, that was charged by the cord, that connects to the wiring, that adheres to the telephone pole, and allows the power of life to be possible in today's day and age.

YOU'LL FIGURE OUT THAT THOSE WIRES ARE WHY YOU don't overheat in 110° temperatures in the dead of summer because it supplies power to your air-conditioning unit. Those ugly hoses and cables are why your coffee machine supplies what you need in that kick-starter cup in the morning and breaking news to catch you up on the world. When you start thinking like that, those wires no longer seem as ugly – they have their own beauty in their absolute necessity.

So, THE TIME IS HERE TO RETRAIN YOURSELF TO SEE the beauty of the sky and omit the noticing of the wires. At a minimum, I suggest everything you see as intrusive probably has a good side. Even your malfunctioning body will have good days. When you're having a bad day, remember all the things you did on that good day and don't let those wires obstruct your view of that pretty sky.

I HOPE MY TRUE STORIES HAVE INSPIRED OTHERS TO navigate and thrive despite MS. Maybe something I've written gives them clues that might help deal with, and in some cases, recover from some of the symptoms they experience. I think it's important to share lessons learned with this ridiculous disease. Through my experiences, you can see how I've evolved to cope with MS.

I'm shaking the trees so you can reach the low hanging fruit. I understand I am oddly built, tenacious to say the least, but know God made me this way for a reason. Maybe this is the reason. Internal to my being is that I see ways out when cornered. I can be relentless in finding a solution. I'm not doing this as a show, it just is and always has been.

So why am I writing this?

I can't help it.

. . .

THAT IS ALSO SOMETHING GOD HAS BUILT ME WITH. I'm never at a loss for vowels, consonants, or certainly metaphors. I'm nudging you here, and I'm doing it with my own proof. You may not execute your own healing exactly the way I have, but If one person gains one line of inspiration from anything I've written, my mission has been successful.

SANDY O.

10

MY MS SECRETS WITHIN

FEB. 18

WE ALL HAVE SO many things that trigger our daily MS symptomatic lives. The numbers I'm giving below are for some of my symptoms. They are obviously my take on what has worked for me. It's not a prescription to do exactly what I've done – it's just to show you how to fight the monster. If you have a pen, by all means, place your own numbers/priorities for things that have worked for you. For the newbies, here's some of my choices that have positively affected my health.

REDUCING STRESS IS A STRONG 1ST CONTENDER.

SLEEP easily comes in at #2. In fact, great sleep also reduces stress. That goes to show you how easy these items can be flip-flopped in their priority.

Proper medication and nutrients to keep symptoms and uncooperating bloodwork in check comes in 3rd.

Being conscious of foods we put down our gullets is the 4th.

Exercise, functional practice, and keeping our bodies moving in general comes in at #5.

The 6th absolute necessity for me is a firm obedience to

ROUTINES.

I'VE BECOME SO METHODICAL IN MY ROUTINES THAT they no longer own me; I own them. That is to say that they have become a part of my natural routine, as opposed to the fact that I have not become a part of *their* routine. We work in absolute synergy – tandem dancers if you will. The beginning of my routines started with my first MS disease modifying therapy (DMT) medicine. It's incredibly important to keep apprised of all risks and side effects of any drug you're on or thinking of going on. After all, you are your best advocate and/or your significant other, if you have cognition impairments.

SO, FOR MY FIRST DMT, IT WAS IN THE PILL FORM. MY prescription told me to take it with breakfast and dinner but the math in that sentence doesn't equate for me. There are 24 hours in a day, last time I checked. I wanted my body to have a chance to dilute the medicine evenly, so I developed my first MS routine by taking the pills every 12 hours. Since that medicine has the potential for gastrointestinal issues (diarrhea and nausea), I found that a packet of Better & Oats Thick & Hearty Blueberry Muffin oatmeal does the trick. I will name things specifically in this story as they were processes of my trial-and-error landing on found successes in product. My opinions within are honest and true arrivals at points where I experimented with my own results. It's not meant to say you should do this, but it is meant to say that arrival at your own points is essential to your own success.

OK, SO I'M UP AT 5AM, I HAVE THE ABOVE-MENTIONED blueberry oatmeal and add blueberries to the mix. In case you don't know, blueberries are excellent for the brain. I found the best blueberries are organic and, in my case, "Driscolls" fit the bill perfectly for both taste, size, and affect. In addition to the above, I usually have 10 ounces of a 25/75 drink mix of Ocean Spray's Cran-Grape mixed with water. The Cran-Grape is good for my neurogenic bladder and the water is good for my neurogenic bowel.

More on that part later.

WE'RE STILL ON BREAKFAST.

I also mix several nuts and seeds in a large Ziploc bag and scoop a palm full to have with my breakfast. That mixture includes walnuts, pecans, sunflower seeds, shelled pistachios, cashews, and sliced almonds. I sift them through a sieve to get as much of the salt off them as possible. I eat them because they're clean proteins – that's better for me than fat, artery clogging proteins. The last thing I have with my breakfast is dark chocolate. If I get the thick bar of Hershey's dark chocolate, I have one square. If I get the thin bar of dark chocolate, I have 1/4 of the bar (3 squares).

Look it up.

Dark chocolate is also excellent for the brain. Please remember, everything in moderation. It just so happens that I love dark chocolate, but I had to switch to eating it for function, not for gluttony. Keeping your weight in check is also a concern with those of us with MS as our mobility slows down and weight gain can soon follow.

OK, I FORGOT TO MENTION AN UNMENTIONABLE.

Before I get up to prepare my breakfast, I must pee. I'm telling you that after years facing multiple deficiencies with that region, I have learned the secret (for me). When I was working,

I could not go! The thing is, I did not know that I had to go or that my bladder was completely full. That, by the way, turned into bladder infections I didn't even know I had. These types of infections have more to do with the fermenting and supplementing of your urine as opposed to the other kind where you wipe the wrong way.

Boy do you know when you have that infection!

It stings and burns.

MS and the buffoonery of nerves disturbs that sensation... at least in my case. There were too many times that I had to attend to meetings, deadlines, work issues to resolve, and expectations of requirements. We had a 6-stall work bathroom. By hearing others with hydraulic force urination, it was all a distraction for me, and I could not go. All that added to my already damaged bladder's nerve wiring that would not let me urinate. Heck, I didn't even know I had a full bladder – that's what a neurogenic bladder can cause. I was also mentally running all night long by making lists on my iPhone of things to do the next day, the next week, month, and year. My brain would never shut up, but my bladder sure did. When you add in what MS already short circuits to the nerve endings affecting bladder and bowel function, the result for me was a continuous problem of sedentary fermenting bladder infections.

THESE ARE COMMON ISSUES WITH MS AND CAN CAUSE exacerbations due to infections which resulted in tons of amassing MS symptoms on my case. I wish I didn't find that out the hard way but, perhaps somebody will preventively learn something from my story earlier than I did. Here's what I found out through very stubborn insisting of my body to perform this very basic function we all take for granted.

First of all...

Shhhh! Lights off!

I can have no distractions – it's just me and the bladder.

Then there's a long slow inhale and exhaling release that I do and hold while I patiently wait for the tingling sensation that allows me to go. In the beginning of my system troubleshooting, what worked for me was the lowering of my head and, for some reason, that allowed for a *zing* in the nerves in my spine and bladder. All I had to do was wait for the familiar tingle that felt like the bladder was about to let me have my way to release said ingredient (pee). I did that for several months and got very good at streamlining the necessary sensation, but part of that action was to allow my innards to settle.

IT'S KIND OF LIKE HOW A WOMAN TAKES HER BRA OFF and her breasts settle – I was allowing that with my bladder. The bladder and possibly the uterus were relaxing and lowering. Ultimately, I had to change how well that worked because the relaxing of my lower innards made it so that I had to urinate too often and sometimes, without control as I'd hurry to the bathroom. I had to adapt that initial process to achieve the same goal, minus allowing my bladder and uterus to lower. I'm offsetting that now by doing more stomach muscle flexing exercises, deep knee bends, and more movements to restore my system. I got so good at voiding my bladder that it can actually growl when emptied, like a hungry stomach growl.

Once I solved the denying voiding anomaly, the sensation of an empty bladder was, and still is, so incredibly satisfying. Now, I take a very full and slow inhale into my lungs while extending my back straight up with my neck and head up too, and then I freeze. I then, very, very slowly let the air out of my lungs and by the time I get to the bottom of that volume of air, it triggers the bladder's wiring and allows me to begin to urinate.

Something very important to note is, just because I start going, doesn't mean I keep going. It often stops several times midstream. Ok...so more inhales and exhales allow for the segmented releases and my patience and strict task attention is required to allow for a full release.

THIS IS A DAILY ROUTINE I MUST KEEP FOR MY health. By the way, I've had two urologists ask me to explain how I overcame the retention of holding urine. Both were men and they don't have the same parts, so they can't feel what I'm saying, but women can physically understand this. Initially, I went from doctors having conversations with me about their remedy to periodically catheterize myself and surgical options! Keep in mind, at that time I was dealing with egregious failure of my hands and dexterity was out of the question. That was a new symptom for me that was directly tied to infections in my bladder I did not know I had. I knew I needed time to figure this one out. Since I was already dealing with the very impacting dexterity issues, I had to work out the details and resolve this issue... and I did!

So far, it has worked for 3 years.

BUT I DIGRESS.

Back then, when breakfast was over, I'd brush my teeth and head back to sleep for another hour or two. My natural second alarm clock were those 10 ounces I drank at breakfast calling on me, so the bladder routine continued.

Now, it's time for coffee. I make my 2 cups worth, and another BIG SECRET is Reese's Cups. If you're a diabetic, obviously sugar's out of the question so regular peanuts do the same trick. I used to be prescribed two docusate pills a day plus MiraLAX to help me go #2. That inability is also an all-too-common MS signature trait.

More of those pesky nerve damage issues.

So, with the coffee and a Reese's cup, within an hour of that routine – all systems are a go! As a result of the above, I do not make outside plans until mission success has occurred. Coffee (caffeine) has a specific function – at least with a woman's bladder. It creates convulsions. So, I'm able to kill two birds with one stone... so to speak.

Wait!

I love birds... I need a new metaphor.

How about this: crush two rocks with one hammer?

Ehh, it's weak but I'll go with it.

NOW, I'M OFF TO THE RACES FOR WHATEVER THE DAY'S limited plans are.

Grocery shopping, minor house cleaning, appointments, or whatever is on my to-do list. More often than not, the tasks are inside and dependent on my energy level.

On to lunch.

If I have a sandwich, it's usually turkey (clean meat), and sometimes with ham (not so clean meat). What lunch usually includes is popcorn. Once I learned it's a fiber, it was game on. I add another glass of water, and together, they aid in the ability to go #2 the next day! The above actions removed my need to be on any stool softeners or laxatives. It's always my goal to get off supplements and do something naturally. My splurge item goes along with my earlier coffee. Having tried all the store brand blueberry muffins, I landed on Brahms blueberry muffins. With those, I don't feel like I'm eating a bowl of sugar, I don't get heartburn from them, and I definitely taste and see the blueberries. To repeat, blueberries are excellent brain food.

Let's proceed on to movement.

. . .

I OFTEN WALK TRACKS IN MY HOUSE BY WALKING FROM one end to the other for 1/2 an hour with my arms punching out, to and fro (with excellent music playing, of course). It helps to offset the treadmill's boring monotony. The goal being to be near my bathroom until the coffee is completely finished having its way with my bladder. I also continue with intentional deep knee bends to pick things up in lieu of bending at the waist since I have a weak lower back. I used to count how many squats I did per day but, what's the point? I just do it and am stronger for having done so. I also bought this adjustable hand grip that is apparently designed for Arnold Schwarzenegger, which is why I have it on its weakest setting. I must keep my hand strength up because that is another failing entity with MS. Furthermore, there is mechanical dexterity taskings to work on my issues as well as keeping hand strength up.

OK, sorry, I got sidetracked.

Back to dinner...

SALAD IT IS... WELL, MOST DAYS. WHILE THAT'S GOOD for me, I do indulge in Ranch dressing. I'm well aware that it is important that I keep some things that may not be the best choice, so I don't become bored with my routine. Minor gluttony, such as ranch, makes me happy. I would imagine it would be pretty hard to maintain my routine if it was all – hard work. So, it's important to give myself a break and splurge on a couple things.

Dinner also includes that modified breakfast drink.

In this case, 1/4 Cran-Grape or prune juice, 1/4 of V-8 pomegranate blueberry drink, and the rest water. Pomegranate has a natural anti-inflammatory nature to it, and I've already explained the beneficial bit about blueberries and how water always helps our hydration to offset the constipation issues caused by MS. I have it with a half of a thin bar of Hershey's dark chocolate. As mentioned before, my online research said that dark chocolate is excellent for the brain, and my cognition is quite good.

I was able to get off my morning vitamin C supplement by adding more vitamin C drinks and foods into my daily repertoire. I still take one at night considering that I am sedentary and unable to drink vitamin C at night since I don't want to brush my teeth at midnight.

THE LAST BIT OF MY DAILY ROUTINE COMES IN THE evening. I often have a cup of green tea at night. I used to drink regular tea, but I switched to green tea once I learned of its benefits to the body. Some other things I switched to was real honey instead of processed sugar. With my green tea I found that I didn't even need the creamer or honey with it, and I can drink it straight. Again, I'm focusing on the gain – not the loss of adding sweet and cream to a healthy drink.

Finally, I happily succumb to my fully encompassing pillows, and sleep very, very soundly. That is a major part of our lives we must adhere to. Sleep when tired – no apologies necessary. Like I said, I live in sync with my routines.

This story has been on my mind for a while as I've run into several people who are currently struggling with many things that I've already found solutions for. Perhaps this story will let people see that there is a way forward and that many of the things with MS are completely solvable with deliberate actions on your part. Good luck, and I hope something in this story proves beneficial to you.

Ode to the routines.

SANDY O.

11

9-11 & MS
VETERANS DAY

I TRIPPED over emotions today that I haven't let pour out of me since the last remembrance of that somber day. My phone reminded me that I have an appointment this morning. I remembered yesterday's news talking about the anniversary today, but the memories did not flood in until later.

I'M AT THE VA'S LABORATORY TO HAVE MY BLOOD drawn and, surprisingly, to have a urinalysis requirement too. The first requirement I am instantly ready for, but not the second one. People with MS learn quickly to use the restroom before they leave the house for anything. So, my bank's coffers are quite empty and sipping water I must do. My focus is on my bladder and nothing else until the proverbial 2 x 4 smacks me in the forehead.

WHAT TIME IS IT?!?!?!

A FULL BLOOD RUSH IN MY BODY REMINDS ME OF THE time frame I'm at. I have full recollection of that day. It's 9:01, the moment of silence should be here in two minutes. I'm not seeing behaviors that would suggest that the silence will actually happen.

That can't be!

I'm in a sea of veterans.

This can't be!

I'm already a woman on the emotional edge, given this day, this offence remembered, and of this world changing event. Life was never the same – how could it be?

ALREADY WITH A FROG IN MY THROAT, I WALK OVER TO the woman at the desk, and I can't speak. I show her on my iPhone the timelines of 9-11. I explain in my cracking voice –

"We're 1 minute away (the 2nd tower's crash). Can you please turn the TV off for a moment of silence?"

"If everyone else agrees with that," she states.

The weight of that sentence instantly suffocates me. She's not going to say anything – it's left up to me.

THE FROG HAS GROWN TOAD SIZED AS I TRY TO address the room.

"Attention everyone, we are less than a minute away from the anniversary of the plane..."

It's at a point I can't talk because I'm crying. I continue.

"...Since the plane hit the twin towers. Does anybody have a problem if we turn the TV off for a moment of silence?"

I am quite emotional, but no one speaks or makes a gesture. Partly out of embarrassment for my lack of control on this very poignant date and time, I take my seat. The woman at the desk takes a minute and starts to turn the TV's volume lower.

. . .

I KNOW SHE CAN'T POSSIBLY KNOW THAT I TAKE THAT as an insult to those who perished. I am trying to get a moment of silence – to have people shift back to that day when the world's axis was shifted. The woman turns the TV back up within a minute, but my tears continue as I know there are four timestamps.

8:46am – the first plane hits the first tower.

9:03am – the second plane hits the second tower.

9:37am – the third plane crashes into the pentagon and the fourth plane's passengers bravely attempted overtaking control, but...

10:03am – it was crashed, by terrorists, in Pennsylvania.

Each one of those actions is a buried very real timeline occasion in my head... in my body.

9-11-2001: I'M IN MY SHOP AT MY BASE. MY BUDDY "Doogan" comes storming out of the office and yells in his thick Georgian drawl.

"AN AIRPLANE JUST CRASHED INTO THE TWIN TOWERS IN NEW YORK CITY!!!"

I freeze.

Everyone is running to the other side of the hangar to get to a TV to see it but I can't move. Slowly I wander into the office. My brain processes it as a biplane –a small plane. "Doogan" comes back screaming.

"ANOTHER PLANE JUST HIT THE SECOND TOWER...IT'S THE GOD DAMN TERRORISTS!!"

THE TUNING FORK PING OF THOSE WORDS I WILL never forget.

My body went into auto drive. I never went to see it on the TV – I knew exactly what I had to do. I called for all my crew to get their asses back to their mechanical work and turn those assets out! This is BIDnes!!! I knew our future... our Wing's future would deploy for this sickness. Turn those wrenches... I only want to see asses and elbows (a maintenance jobbin'out [balls-to-the-wall] term). Instantly, we're all focused on the purpose of every gig we clear, every nut we tighten, every rig we pin...etc. We don't care how many hours it takes...we just perform with so much vigor you could pick it up on a Richter scale.

THE BUZZ OF THE WORKDAY ENDS AND I PICK UP MY child from the daycare.

I'm in a daze.

My daughter is very perceptive and is looking at me quite perplexed. Heck, I'm perplexed with the world and myself at this moment, so I understand her odd expression. I know she's reading everything I've experienced on my face.

We get home.

Finally, and quite reluctantly, I turn the TV on. Anyone from my generation knows where they were on 9-11. The sights I'm seeing slam me to my knees.

Dear Lord... Dear Lord.

My daughter gingerly approaches me and stands before me. She's blocking my view from what my eyes can't unsee. I reach for her and pull her close. I'm peeking over her shoulder at evil personified.

"What have I done... what have I done?"

I brought this child into *this world*. What have I done?

Nothing is guaranteed anymore. All my thoughts go to, what life is ahead of her?

What have I done?

The air... breathing is different. The ground beneath my feet feels strange. Space and time are now warped, and I see the devil in the flesh on the news footage that accelerates and never seems to end.

RETURNING TO TODAY – MY FACE, NOW RED AND blotchy from crying, is inexplicably in view of my laboratory waiting compadres. I'm finally ready to provide that second delivery requirement having sipped water through my tears.

With my head down and tears still dripping, I placed my specimen in the tenant's tray. I forgot to mention while I was waiting for contents to deliver said package, I called the VA director's number and got his secretary. In tears, and inaudibly crying I say,

"8:46, 9:03, 9:37, and 10:03 are 9-11's significant times. Isn't there supposed to be moments of silence?"

She says, I don't know.

I ask if the director is in – he's not. I think I said something like, please tell him... and had to hang up from crying.

AFTER LEAVING THE LAB, I WALK THROUGH THE VA, tears in tow, and stop at the greeter's help desk. I collect myself with a few deep breaths and asked the men if the VA exercises moments of silence (I'm already crying and having difficulty talking) for the 9-11 remembrance and honoring. One of them states he thinks the flag is at half-staff. I take a big breath.

I do understand there's so many campaigns and deaths related to them. The VA can't possibly recognize all of them. Those prior to my service escapes me at present, so I understand, but it still hurts. As my voice breaks up from crying, I say,

"This is my generation's Kennedy moment."

With that, I turn and fade away towards the exit... tears still in tow.

. . .

I GET TO MY CAR.

Actually, I rushed to my car knowing what time it was. As my tail end hits the car seat, it's 9:37 – the 3rd plane had just hit the Pentagon and another full-on episode of recollection of this day ensues. I thank God that I made it to my car where I can sit in silence in the company of my eye's salty water.

Soon after, I proceed on my ride home. The radio's still off and I'm floating down the road with my unfortunate memories. It's much like a dream where you're traveling, but you're not walking... just floating from scene to scene. Traffic slows, and I see now that the train is stationary across the tracks. For once, I welcome it as an unintentional moment of silence. I'm quite alone in my interpretation as I watch a series of cars immediately start their U-turns to divert what they know will be a long train crossing.

WE HAVE JUST MINUTES TO GO BEFORE THE 4TH PLANE is heroically overtaken (attempted), by passengers but was ultimately crashed in Pennsylvania by the terrorist. Frustrated, I leap out of the car to the closest commercial truck. I knock on his door and he lowers the window.

Again, with a sobering voice, I say, "Can you help me?"

He says yes.

I ask him, "Can you get on your CB radio and let everybody know that at 10:03, it's a significant time stamped with the crash of the 4th plane on 9-11."

His face contorts to empathy as he says he has no radio and I just melt.

No words.

I have no words for trying to inform everybody of this date and time stamp of where they are and what needs to be remembered. I wobble (MS signature walk), back to my car, unbelievably somber and feeling defeated.

THE FIREFIGHTERS, THE POLICE OFFICERS, THE emergency first responders, and I'm sure the countless citizens trying to help co-workers... all HEROS.

They are resoundingly with me today.

Maybe it's not all my tears. There's so many – I must be channeling them and shedding their tears as well. Their loved ones left behind, their stations remembering their brothers and sisters.

This makes sense to me.

I'm mourning the day and living the sorrow for myself as well as being a vessel for other's tears. That explains the quantity pouring out of my eyes. What surfaces in my thoughts is that life goes on. It's with that premise that I am faced with what I only can know. I have arrived at this point repeatedly, daily, hourly, and by the minute.

I HAVE MULTIPLE SCLEROSIS.

It likes to proceed forward, and I strive to retrieve backwards. It's a tough subject and people disappear quickly from your life. Believe me, if I could walk away from this disease, I would. I hold nobody accountable for doing the same.

I don't want this disease to stick around.

I don't want to deal with the tic-tac-toe game it likes to play. All X's and no O's. It plays a dirty game.

If you can walk away, I can't blame you. You know why? Because life goes on.

Just like 9/11 and people continuing with their daily lives – that is precisely what I must do every day despite this piece of shit disease.

SANDY O.

. . .

SO, NO JUDGMENT ON ANY OF THOSE WHO WERE NOT in the same emotional place I was at during 8:46, 9:03, 9:37, or 10:03 today. The same goes for no judgment to anyone who walks away from me not wanting to deal with the same disease I HAVE to deal with every day.

Because... life goes on.

SANDY O.

12

SHIT PIE

OCT. 31

My Sarcastic Recipe:

Prep with daughter's late-night return from work and commence to conversation till... ohhhh, dark 30.

Start with 3 hrs. of sleep.

Add in concerns about missing tomorrow's appointment.

Set timer for early wake-up.

Sprinkle with exhaustion.

Gradually add in that the dogs need to go outside, corralled back inside, and then fed.

Combine thoroughly with too much to do and not enough time to do it.

Wash the wobbly carcass in a hurried lukewarm shower where you feel pressed for time.

Whip up a failed attempt to dry hair minus showing of natural cowlick.

Bring slowly to a boil an unsuccessful attempt to put on earrings and makeup. Wash and re-rinse!

Heat up oatmeal breakfast so it readily fries my already agitated tooth's nerves and hit it from the left with a cold drink of Cran-Grape and water for perfect lightning bolts of electrocution.

Knead together firmly the cleaning of teeth with further rounds of torture from brush contact and cold sink water for an extra mind-boggling series of jolted pain.

Insert legs into my damn doctor's appointment stockings!

Remove stockings!

Dabble with a panicked rush for time (still sportin' 3 hrs. of sleep).

Keep watching that clock... it's still ticking.

Pressure's building!

Lightly sauté an attempt to Pee. Friggin' Peeeee ALREADY! BM!... something... GIVE ME SOMETHING!!!

Cover ingredients with STRONG pins and needles!

Bake in pressure which adds finite dexterity buffoonery!

Add 2 Nostrils of congestion with leaking by-products.

Boil in secondary swelling of gums (i.e., excruciating nerve pain).

Mix thoroughly with gut wrenching screams of frustration and defeat!

Dress the stress-ball in my tan coat. The pig skin's too tight for the sausage... Crap...this is my daughter's tan coat! Youngin', come rescue me out of this thing!

Additional vats of more pathetic salty tears commence.

Stir ingredients for heightened volatility in crockpot at highest setting.

Finally, cook for 2 hours in a strong dousing of tears until burnt, and voila...

There you have a perfectly baked MS SHIT PIE.

Enjoy... *NOT*!!

Serve slices on a shingle and grab a fork! All slices feed 1 MS patient having a very bad morning.

Fuck you, Halloween!

Sandy O.

13
CANTILEVER
FEB. 5

I'M GOING to painstakingly explain what that title means to those of you who are not mechanically inclined, or at least mechanically curious. Once you figure out the yin and yang of cantilever, your MS lives will be so much more enhanced. Moreover, everything that tells you no, can be turned into a mission to defy and conquer.

Cantilever is a process I used repeatedly in my prior mechanical career. It's the seesaw effect where one side is pushed up, and the other side must go down – weights and/or strength being equal counterparts. I'll except the help from a cane or a walker in the beginning of an MS snafu, but will defy any obstacle by finagling another way forward.

So, let's begin from the day's start.

I ROLL THE BLANKETS OFF ME AND MOVE MY encasing pillows to the other side of the bed. As I bring my legs straight up, I swing them down in the counterbalance position and place my right hand on the nightstand to push off for the left upright action. My legs dropping, catapults me upwards, and the right hand is pushing me directionally to the left. Then it's a trip to the restroom where even lowering myself to the commode also requires counterbalance. Thank goodness I have a very small master bathroom because it really does come in handy. With that small bathroom comes a small commode. Of note for me is that a small commode and a small toilet seat makes for a very uncomfortable frequent trip.

I needed to pursue a more accommodating *landing zone*.

So, I shopped at my local hardware store. If I get a longer/higher *butt receptacle*, it will take up too much room in that very confined space. After patrolling the options, I confirmed that it would, indeed, take up far too much geography in my already minuscule en suite.

Still digging for a solution, I found a wall of just toilet seats. Low and behold, I found the one I wanted and needed. I chose one with a split as I have friends who visit who have to catheterize and that split option provides them the access they need.

The salesperson tried to convince me that a larger toilet was necessary for those longer split seats and I said, *not so fast*. They all have universal attachments that will fit any toilet – it fit mine perfectly... sort of. The connectivity (bolts), fit perfect but the shape was over the size of my small round toilet. Still, the bowl's structure was under the seat, so it still worked. It also helps my comfort level, my pocketbook, and in lifting the toilet seat when cleaning it. Now, there's just one more counterbalance requirement in this action.

For balance reasons, mechanical cantilever is required in the dissent to my low toilet. I place my hand on the wall in front of me and push off it gently to aim for the *target area*.

Success...

I did not fall, and I hit the landing zone perfectly. So far, that's 3 checkmarks for me:

Getting out of bed without falling

Successfully descending to the frequent spot

Adding to my comfort level...my way!

Now to the next solved speed bump.

So as not to scare the neighbors, it's time to get dressed.

I broke my arm recently which means this already inflicted body has an injury to compensate for. Not to worry – this is a fixed card game I know all too well...

We're back to finagling.

I hook my bra first and then slip it on. I had to figure that one out right away because it takes two hands to clip a bra, so with one arm in a sling and the other doing the clipping... problem solved! I lean right on my bed as I raise my left leg and insert it into my all too frequently worn ugly stretch pants. Since I also hurt my right leg in that arm breaking trip and fall, lifting it is no easy task. I drop the pants to the floor and can scoop my right leg into the hole's opening. Now all that's left is to lift the pants to my waist and I can do that with one hand. This is all done by shoring my body up against my bed's mattress.

If the above is precluded by a shower, that task is absolutely loaded with sets of cantilever and centering necessities. My shower is also extremely small, a space paramount to my safety. It has one of those doors that closes which is also essential as I'm sure if it was a shower curtain, I would've fallen through it easily. My right hand's placement on the shower's opening allows me to lean right and pull to facilitate the lifting of my left leg over the 4-inch entrance's lip. Equally important as I proceed through, is pushing off the same right hand to now bring the right leg over that same threshold.

Pushing, pulling, and leaning are a part of my daily life now. I don't even think about it anymore – it just comes naturally.

AT NO TIME DO I STAND IN THE SHOWER WITHOUT MY body, an arm, hand, or knee touching either a wall or a shelf. That's because I am leaning over to get my shampoo or reaching up to grab my scrunchie. It's especially prudent to either lean, brace, or push/pull in the choreography of my shower. If my wet eyes are closed, it's very dangerous for me because my center becomes lost. I'm sure you've heard of people explaining how disorienting it is during an earthquake when they don't have a solid footing. That's very similar to when my eyes have to be closed. I know it's not technically a counterbalance when I'm talking about centering. However, I have to know where I am to orient myself, hence my hand, arm, knee or body needing to touch a wall or shelf. The exiting of the shower has all the same markings of entering so I won't repeat them.

We'll move on to another normality for me.

ABOUT A MILLION TIMES A DAY, I HAVE TO MOVE THE towel I cut in half and placed on the floor to deal with the dog's slobber after drinking their water. Any liquid on the floor is a huge slipping and falling danger for me. So, I have to scoot that towel back in place or else! Keeping my left foot on the carpet, I have to put my hand on the corner of the wall, push on it and use the right leg to scoot that towel back into place on the linoleum kitchen floor. Additionally, if I have to move something heavy from the stove or refrigerator to the sink, my hip or my other hand is on the kitchen counter to oppose that weight.

That is cantilever.

ANOTHER EXAMPLE IS, I HAVE A GIANT DOG THAT likes to stop right in front of me in confined areas as if to say, 'please pet me for the billionth time'. Much like weaning a baby off the teet, I sometimes have to walk around her.

Do you know how hard it is to walk around a giant in a small space?

I have to reach my hand out and push on the wall or the arm of the sadly unused treadmill as a counterbalance for that action to go around this giraffe of a dog.

LASTLY, MY GARAGE IS A TIGHT SPACE SO EVEN getting to my car door requires me to ricochet from my car to the wall as I navigate the small channel to my front door.

You know how us MSers usually walk with our legs wide out like a two-year-old learning to balance walking?

It doesn't work well when the space is tight, hence my ricocheting back and forth.

If you're not using yourself as a counterbalance, I hereby grant you full autonomy to take the bull by the horns. It's not only empowering, but also confidence building, which quite a bit of us actually need.

For the most part, I don't stop anything – I just figure out another way. I get frustrated more than the average bear and need to figure out that which obstructs my functionality. I could list scores of other things that mean the same, but I hope you get the point.

. . .

SANDY O.

I'VE SEEN THE SCARED FACES ON THE FIRST-TIME
support group meeting attendees. You can actually see them
looking and fearing of their own future's demise through the
various states of health of other MSers in the room.

I'm here to tell you, that's not the case.

You're seeing people who've been through things minus
medicine, minus physical therapy transformations, and some
who are not built with the tenacity to overcome.

It's NOT your future.

I have learned so many pivotal things from organizations like
the NationalMSSociety.org, the Cando-MS.org, and MSworld.org
(love their chat room). There are so many things out there to
both help you, enlighten you, include you, and empower you.
It's very freeing, and very motivating for me to keep up with the
latest and greatest – it's my livelihood.

Everything's an *angle to the dangle* in my world.

SO GO GET YOU SOME!!! IT'S ALL THERE FOR THE
taking.

SANDY O.

1 4

MS'S OPTICAL ILLUSIONS
FEB. 8

"YOU LOOK like you're doing so good! You look Great!"

WHAT?!!!

I let those words roll off my back now, but it was really hard to take, just a few short years ago. Comments like that force you to think of why you're *not* doing great. It makes you start to assess what's really wrong with your body as opposed to what people see.

You may have been perfectly engaged in work, not thinking about MS and then those comments happen. It puts you right back into the sickening world of MS because you know better.

If my coworkers only knew – everything they saw was an MS optical illusion.

I HAVE HAD TO LIVE WITH THE ODDITIES OF WHAT THE other side of the world looks like with the many ridiculous antics of MS. I've always had a visual of what it would look like if people could see what I experience 'below the waterline'.

In the cover, you will see that visual.

It's only some of what is below the waterline, but I think

you'll get the point after reading the story. I knew what I wanted it to look like so I drew a sketch, and I knew what that would entail.

THE HALOGEN LIGHT MUST BE FLASHED ON THE ridiculous MS carcass. There will be no secrets to hold me back from this disease. FYI, the image does not capture all of my symptoms as there's only so much space. Further, not all the symptoms shown were suffered at one time.

I suspect that many are induced by my own actions that agitate the disease. Things like, not having proper sleep for two nights in a row is a done deal. Having too much stress is a further antagonist to my symptomology. Exposure to heat is brutal to my body – in fact, it's intolerable. Partaking in salty foods, sugars, or just not eating healthy are also red carpet invites to the disgusting things you'll hear about here.

TO BE TRUTHFUL, I'M THE ONLY ONE WHO KNOWS exactly what the disgusting, exasperating truth is below the waterline. So, hold onto something – here comes the flashlight.

Just like 90% of an iceberg is below water, so too is our MS lives. The world sees the 10% of me, and I wanted that 90% articulated visually.

The upper image is the normal looking person, the 10% the public sees, and the 90% (MS symptoms) contrast below water... the iceberg effect. The *thing* below that deep gray murky water needed to be illustrated. I think any other person would want that world hidden, but I find that everything you keep to yourself becomes a tool used against you.

With respect to the artist's interpretation, the cover is but a fraction of what's below my actual waterline. Besides, it's probably TMI for a large part of the audience.

It's time to open the curtains on the monsters below deck – a visual for the invisible symptoms I've lived with off and on for decades.

FATIGUE IS COMMON WITH MS. FOR A WHILE THERE I was prescribed B12 since my levels were very low. It's kind of like operating in syrup where it feels like even picking up your arms or bringing your drinking glass to your mouth can be a struggle. After all, we all have bad days. So many of the symptoms will reflect what they're like on those bad days. My B12 levels recovered but I do have an occasional episode. I now rarely take a small measure of B12 and it usually kickstarts me back to normal. I don't have to do that but maybe once a quarter as I started filling in my diet with natural sources of B12.

Proceeding on, there's a difference between dizziness and vertigo.

ONE TIME, WHILE LAUGHING AND TURNING TO GET out of my bed, it felt like somebody violently slammed me back onto my pillow. I froze because I didn't understand what happened. Then, I slowly tried to get up again and I got the same sensation of being slammed back onto my bed.

Long story short, it immediately caused me to vomit nonstop. I couldn't move or open my eyes, or it got worse. A 911 call and a rescue were required...

It was my first bout with vertigo.

It stayed with me for a while and came back at work where I had to be physically walked to my car and driven home. I'd rather have dizziness every day of my life instead of one more episode of vertigo.

It's a brain malfunction for sure, and there are more.

. . .

SANDY O.

An MRI shows my brain and spine have all the usual icky lesions of MS simmering in a pot. Another disfunction is my upper lip area gets moving sensations like there's wiggling worms in it. I remember being at work, fearing that people could actually see the twitching of what felt like meal worms beneath my nose, descending to my upper lip.

I kept grabbing at my face to hide my secret from the onlookers. That symptom broadened to twitters and insane itches in my face. That condition is called facial myokymia. It occasionally stops by for a day or two.

Another usual tandem cohort with MS is optic neuritis. I was the raffle winner on that one too.

My work's AC broke... again, and I became extremely overheated. On top of that, I was under high pressure which created a visual affect with the patterned floor. It looked like it was shaking, and focusing my eyes was out of the question. Concerned coworkers convinced me to go to the ER to rule out a stroke.

What was the line from that movie, Animal House?

Oh yeah – "Thank you, may I have another" – as the sorority brothers smack the pledge's derrière...very apropos!

The episode fried an optic nerve leading to the diagnosis of optic neuritis. I remember there was a shadow seen in the center of my eye's view, kind of like a cold window having that fog on it.

Sticking to the eyes for a minute, double vision as well as a bout of esotropia were impatiently in line for their turn. Some happened with no visual indications to the bystander, but that last one had my eyeball turning inward, and everybody saw it. I was diagnosed with esotropia and it took about six months, but it did recover itself. A coworker devised a mask blocking out the affected eye to replace my drug store bought black patch. I got a kick out of that and I appreciated somebody seeing the humor in that which I could not control.

Here's another doozy!

I REMEMBER BEING OVERWHELMED BY THE SENSATION of an overtightened, medieval iron – like a brace around my abdomen – on my bra line to be exact. I could not catch my breath and I was so incredibly uncomfortable no matter what position I was in. That symptom directly correlates to the rather large lesion in my spine. I've heard other MSers refer to that as the "MS hug". Well, it doesn't feel like a hug to me, it feels like a torture device and it comes back from time to time.

Now to my hands, but that's a paragraph in and of itself.

THERE WAS A TIME THAT I NOT ONLY LOST THE capability to hold a utensil, but I couldn't feel anything in my hands. That meant, I dropped everything and had to stop driving. On top of that is the pins and needles feeling, or paresthesia, to use the medical term. I also couldn't put my fingers together in a line, like to articulate the number four.

It was weird.

I couldn't collapse my fingers to touch each other or cup them like you do when you brush your teeth and rinse your mouth out with water. When those were my symptoms a few years ago, I had to be hospitalized for a relapse... new damage.

A few days of Methylprednisolone was my daily IV requirement and it worked.

To continue with my hands, when my adrenaline is high or if I'm overheated, I get a very weird sensation. It's like a small ice cream scooper has dug out chunks of flesh from my fingers and I can feel the divots. I find myself rubbing my fingers together for the pseudo sensation of scoops of missing flesh. It's a thing but it doesn't own me.

Now we're headed south... pun intended!

I WAS VERY DISRESPECTED BY A TALENTED BUT immature man I worked with. He did something that hadn't been done to me despite having been in a male working environment for over 25 years.

While explaining the work requirements for a very urgent situation to a team of relevant people, he was standing behind me in my blind spot. He wet his finger and stuck it in my ear. I want to reiterate that I've been respected in a world not typical for a female for decades. My instant reflex was to swat at whomever was to the rear.

While he laughed and got others to laugh with him, I screamed.

"Oh no... Oh No... OH NO!"

I knew how bad it was right away.

It was the most excruciating pain because that swatting motion caused my bicep tendon to tear. The intense pain from that action brought on such a severe battery of symptoms, even the urgent care doctor had never heard of it.

MY ENTIRE CROTCH WENT COMPLETELY NUMB instantly! It felt like my anatomy was plastic like a doll's body. It made all my itchy bits alien to me – a mannequin of sorts. A whole rush of symptoms ensued from that one heinous, disrespectful action from a clown needing attention. I lived with that eerie sensation for several months.

Those of us with MS are already afflicted in our nervous system with various short circuitries (my word) – uncalled for things, like a loss of sexual sensation and/or desire. MS does that to many of us.

And since we're in that quadrant, let's talk about the bladder and the bowel.

UNTIL MY UROLOGIST TEAM PROVED VIA AN ultrasound that I actually had a full bladder, I had no idea and certainly no sensation that it was full. So many of my MS symptoms were due to the result of retaining urine... sort of a fermenting that caused infections I had no idea I had.

An inability to go #2 was also part of the new sickening boardgame of MS. Medically speaking, they're called a neurogenic bladder and bowel. Not to worry though because I've figured out resolutions for both those problems myself.

I was given medicines in the beginning to remedy both actions but found a natural way to relieve said transactions. It's important to note that the medications upfront are very helpful as you get bombarded with ridiculous things. Until you have time to sort them out, the medication can get you over the hurdles. Some conditions, I'm sure, cannot be figured out in the tenacious way I pursue them, so medication in the long run may be necessary depending on what you're diagnosed with.

CONTINUING IN THE SAME AREA IS ANOTHER profound symptom.

This one is with me even today and I have yet to solve it... but I will. All good things take time.

You know how a baboon has a completely inflamed blown-up, red, irritated, grotesque-looking butt when it's in heat?

That is the visual for what I feel and why I cannot sit on anything that isn't memory foam, and even then, not for long.

I used to lug my portable cushion around with me at work because it was so brutal! It's not just my butt that feels like it's three times bigger than it actually is – that blowtorched, swollen, burning, inflaming mess runs all the way down the back of my thighs. Of course, it magnifies it, and I mean, very much magnifies it, in the heat or with my adrenaline so I have to be careful.

Sorry, I'll get off the central region to give you a break. Let's move onto the limbs.

MY ARMS AND LEGS SUFFER FROM PINS AND NEEDLES too.

It's like very dense pins and needles vibrating in and out.

Remember that toy that has needles poking out where kids put their hands on it to make an impression of their handprint on the backside?

Well, it feels like I'm the game... and the needles are protruding through my body. My feet have the same sensations but that's not all. Imagine that you're barefoot and you're walking on rocks, but you're blindfolded and don't see the rocks. Your first instinct is to pick your foot up from that weird bulging rock sensation. On the bottom of my feet, it literally felt like I had these huge 1-inch boils that protruded, affecting how I stepped or walked. It was another pseudo sensation that felt so real that it would force me to look at my feet to make sure they weren't actually there.

Well, they weren't there, hence the word pseudo. It's often still with me, but it's almost like my mind reformatted it to a more flattened effect that's easier for me to tolerate. In fact, I insist on walking barefoot most of the time because it feels more real than when I have shoes on.

The last thing I want to talk about is quite prevalent with MS and that's balance.

. . .

FOR SOME REASON, ONE LEG DOES NOT WANT TO listen and lags behind in the execution of walking.

Like in marching...

Left, right,

Left, right.

Well, the faulty wiring is more like – left *half-right*, left *half-right*.

It's just another ridiculous thing that can go on with this autoimmune disease. I take things one at a time and I'm doing pretty darned good right now. Anything that opposes me and denies me a basic necessity will eventually get my full attention. Many I've solved, but several are still with me from time to time, or even constantly. I'm not prone to succumb and I've got a mean cerebral right hook which I use against MS all the time.

TAKE THINGS ON, ONE AT A TIME, AND START TO associate if you or your surroundings are causing anything that triggers your symptomology. Like I said, I have figured out so many things and have changed behaviors to offset them accordingly. It proved very beneficial to be prescribed things that gave me a kickstart to figure out *'the this and the that'* of what was going on.

I've been successful in winning over many of the medications. I do take supplements, but with an exception to one, they're all my choice. The doctor is right with the D3 and I'm religious about taking that twice a day. You're pretty much not going to catch me in the sun for long so a D3 supplement is very important in my case. I don't have everything solved but I plan that I will.

I'm predominantly winning the fight.

. . .

SANDY O.

ONE LAST COMMENT, AND I HOPE IT MEANS
something different the second time you hear it.
  "You look like you're doing so good! You look Great!"
  Yeah, What*EVER*...

SANDY O.

15

MY QUOTA IS 1 – MURPHY OBJECTS!

DEC. 14

MS ALWAYS COMES with its own line of arsenal. I can talk non-stop about the daily flavor of inflictions. Anything from fatigue, an uncooperative bladder or bowel, pins and needles, dexterity and gait buffoonery... Etc.

For the sake of my argument, I'm going to count the "snowflakes" of symptomology as 1... MS. That's my quota of things to deal with. Again, I say, my quota is 1.

Coming in through the out-door, is Murphy.

MURPHY'S LAW COULD GIVE A RATS PATOOTIE WHAT your quota is.

Case in point:

Just in the last couple of weeks, a neighbor's dog broke into my next-door neighbor's yard – for about the 10th time! The dog is now next to my fence, indicated by the warning, frenzied barks of my dogs. They're going nuts with the large husky in the wrong yard. Given my next-door neighbor recently had bone surgery, he's not aware that, not only is this dog in his yard again, but it's nose-to-nose with his geriatric, almost blind little dog. So now I'm not only worried about his old dog, but I am also worried that my giant dog will fly over the fence since she's grown to giraffe sized (new 6-foot fence now installed). Add into the equation that I know my next-door neighbor is not quite mobile, so I text him.

"THAT HUSKY IS IN YOUR YARD AGAIN – RIGHT UP next to your dog."

Two seconds after that text, that intruder Husky literally strolls into his cracked open patio door.

Text #2:

"She just went into your house!"

Obviously, I'm worried that he would be caught off guard, but he comes to the back door and does the switch, getting the Husky out and bringing his little dog in. I asked if he would like me to go inform the neighbors again and he says yes.

So off I go.

THROUGH MY HOUSE AND OUT MY FRONT DOOR, I begin to walk over there. I stopped between my house and my next-door neighbors to pet the dogs over the fence and try to calm them down.

I continue to the Husky owner's house.

As I get to his stone protruding walkway, something denies me that last step.

Oh no!

Whatever it was that halted my left foot has denied me that last step and sent me careening onto my left side. What a slow-motion, horrifying descent to that stone protruding walkway. My left shoulder hit the rock pavement first and I heard it crack! The second impact was my ribs being rounded out by the landing pressure. In tandem with that was my head snapping left and hitting that walkway. Last, but not least, was another bull's-eye smack-dab crunch of my left hip! I knew how bad it was when it happened, and I had no air to appropriately scream.

ALL I CAN GET OUT, IN MY INABILITY TO MOVE, WAS pain, a struggle for air, and an agonizing moan. The neighbor across the street had visitors standing in the street who saw the whole thing and definitely heard my moans. As I'm writhing in agony, he says,

"I'm going to call 911."

The next part actually made my psyche chuckle despite the brutal physical place I was in.

He says to 911, "AN OLD LADY FELL..."

Have you ever tried not to laugh while you're wrenched in torturous pain? A bruised ego I can deal with, but it actually hurt more to *not* laugh. Granted, I looked like a hot mess with my $1 estate sale men's oversized red plain T-shirt on, my ugly grey oversized shorts, and my pillow head, need-a-shower, icky hair inside a baseball cap.

OF COURSE, he thinks I'm an old lady. I look quite forgettable today. I mean no disrespect to women of maturity, it's just a millennial's use of the word I'm referring to.

He said something to me before emergency responders arrived that was like a warm blanket.

"Would you like me to pray for you?"

How beautiful a sentence that was. He was the technical first responder – here comes the second.

TWO AMBULANCES, A FIRETRUCK, PARAMEDICS AND A very, very disinterested homeowner showed up.

I shrieked out, "I was only coming to tell you your dog got

out again. She's in the neighbor's yard and he just had surgery so he couldn't come over himself!"

He says, "Oh, she's out," very matter-of-factly.

He motions as if he's going to go and retrieve his dog. That's the only thing I could see him acknowledge – certainly not my pain. By the way, I'd already asked him for his phone number, so I don't have to keep walking over to tell him when his dog escapes, but he never obliged. There's homeowners and then there's neighbors. There's a distinct difference between the two.

Eventually, with no questions asked by me, that same neighbor turned a leaf and did pass me his phone number. I did rescue his dog scores of other times.

No hard feelings.

So, here I am and here we are, ER bound!

Ahhhh, the bumps!

Ahhhh, this idiot is blowing up my veins trying to start an IV.

She's ruptured them from her repeated ignorance!!! She needs more schooling!!!! I have straw veins... any phlebotomist can throw a dagger from across the room, and they'll be successful with me.

That is, except this newbie!

That's all I need is more agony, on top of agony, on top of bumps, on top of what the F's! I hope you're counting because none of these series of events equates to my quota of 1! Murphy's Law has the friggin' mic... AGAIN!

I'm in the ER and surrounded by an audience of bewildered, young people who seem to have never experienced someone in intense, writhing pain before. I know they've heard or said plenty of four-letter words before, but I have a PhD in them. Since I'm in exceptional pain, they're quite pronounced. I can't concentrate on their indifferent expressions – I'm in far too much agony! The Physician's Assistant (PA) presents himself and he gets my vernacular right away – *a brother from another mother*, for sure. I like a man who speaks in facts, not mushy poor you, head patting gestures.

Fast forward – CAT scans and x-ray after x-ray from a tenant who doesn't realize there's a friggin' human being on the table!

HEEEY DUDE, don't grab my arm!!

Don't twist me or jam wedges under me – WARN me first! TELL ME what you're going to do or need, and I'll move it because EVERYTHING HURTS!!!!

Right now, my tears are unstoppable because he's hurting me more.

OH, BY THE WAY, THE GURNEY THEY'RE ROLLING ME around on has a square wheel. You've gotta be friggin' kidding me!

Ouch, Ouch, OUCH!!

All in all, my humerus bone was fractured completely through and shifted, and my ribs are bruised and sore. I got a concussion, and my hip is massively bruised from that protruding stone walkway. I also suspect there's torn tendons because I've had that before, and I know what it feels like. They cut everything off me to get to what they needed to get to. On comes the sling and swaddling brace.

Owwww!

Even the nurses struggle with this one as it's not a normal sling. This one is made of foam and quite cumbersome to completely stabilize any movement from my fractured humerus bone.

Is anybody out there still counting?

Let me help you – IT'S NOT "1"!

. . .

THEY RELEASE ME AND I HAVE TO WAIT NINE DAYS TO
see the bone surgeon. That means, I can't open anything, and
my ribs are so sore I can't even get out of bed by myself. I can't
shower, or squeeze toothpaste on my toothbrush. I can't make
my oatmeal, coffee, feed the dogs, drive... Etc. Don't even get me
started on trying to get a sock or a shoe on, or any kind of
clothing for that matter. My daughter stepped up to the plate in
a way that surprised me. She took off from both of her jobs and
was obviously concerned for my state of *not* well-being.

So, back to the title.

Knowing what my internally prescribed quota is, made this
landslide of events insurmountable. I know I should just be
hunky-dory and take life as it hits me, but I'm not wired that
way. It's been like the olden days of a 15 round heavy weight
bout in the ring with Muhammad Ali.

Murphy's Law and I are the boxers though.

While trying to help me, my daughter said something to me
that gave me plenty to think about.

"WHY DON'T YOU JUST LET ME DO IT, MOM?"

I'm so stubborn that even though I asked for her help, it
destroys me to not be able to do it myself. So, I try to do that
which I've asked her to do and it's frustrating for her. My brain is
counting the number of denials of function being thrown at me
by these injuries, and I'm used to being a bow wave against
anything that opposes my functionality. In this scenario
however, I am seeing how my stubbornness in a very difficult
time is affecting somebody who is trying to be there for me.

WOW!

I just realized this story has changed from how Murphy's Law takes over from what you think is your quota of things to deal with is, to a reminder to me of how difficult it must be for somebody providing support.

I must adapt to accepting help when I need it. I thought I already did that, but this injury proved that I'm not done learning that lesson. As if I have a right to pick my own quota, I realize this is not a script I get to write. I can try and set my life up so that things don't happen, but there's that Murphy's Law we all have to deal with.

MY QUOTA IS 1, OR SO I THOUGHT.

I guess the real question is, what is *His* quota? What lesson does *He* say *He* wants you to learn or somebody else to learn from helping you? I think the recent unfortunate mishap's lesson had to do with receiving help when needed and lending myself to the lessons the support partner is learning through helping me... you.

QUOTA, SCHMOTA. I NEED TO FIND MY CRAYONS AND start coloring. As in, shut up and color.

GET IT?

SANDY O.

16

MY NEW FULL DAY

AUG. 21

GEEZ!

I can't sleep tonight – legs are kicking. I have to remember what I ate that had salt or sugar, too close to bedtime. AC's crankin' but I'm still hot, that is, until I kick off the blankets, and then I'm cold.

Blankets off,

Blankets on,

Flip to the left,

Flip to the right.

The little beagle has no choice but to join the choreography and exhales in frustration.

Screw this!

I'm up early for my usual oatmeal breakfast. Normally, I would be back an hour later, but a repeat of the Antiques Roadshow is on... stayin' up!

TODAY'S 2ND WAKE UP IS AT 8AM, THUS BEGINS MY workday, so to speak.

First off, I'm tired. MS already wears me out quickly, but a bad night's sleep is a cherry on top – and a rotten one at that. Dogs galore want outside, so I must get dressed and oblige. Out I go with them, pooper picker-upper in hand, and it's already too darned hot outside! Yet another depletion of energy to start my MS full day.

I QUIT COFFEE A FEW DAYS AGO BECAUSE I'M NOT thrilled with the convulsions caffeine has on my female plumbing.

So, here's the tally so far:

Bad night's sleep

Ridiculously hot temperatures

No coffee

That's called a triple negative, even despite MS. I've been procrastinating on my bed linens. I remove them and put them all in the wash. While they're cleaning, I'm inundated with high pitched squeaks and several pairs of eager eyes staring me down, so it's toy time.

THERE ARE FOUR DOGS IN MY HOUSE RIGHT NOW:

My 17-year-old lab, my daughter's 2-year-old miniature beagle (who I wrote about in an earlier story called "A Cure for Couch-I-Tus"), an adopted giant 8-month-old Anatolian Shepherd mixed with Greyhound or Great Dane, and a Terrier mix I am babysitting.

My lack of energy will absolutely not do for these dogs. Well, the old lab just watches the show.

So, the squeaky toys, braids of rope, and bouncy balls become a throwing tug-of-war/Olympic playing morning routine.

It's exhausting.

By now, I would've had coffee but nooooo... I gave it up three days ago! Back to my MS full day.

IF I'M GOING TO GET ANYTHING ON MY GROCERY LIST, I'd better do it early. It's a short distance to the store. I'm walking the aisles like a drunk person as I grab my carriable-sized items. Then, I stop by the store right down the street for more oatmeal and blueberry muffins.

Oh, I forgot to confess... guess what I bought at the grocery store...

A can of coffee.

Don't tell anyone.

I decided I was already working with a triple negative today and still had things to do... and blah blah blah ... and uphill both ways ... and the sky is falling... Etc. (intentional run-on sentence).

I know, I know...excuses, excuses, but... *what had happened was*... I'M TIRED!!!!

I need COFFEE TODAY!!!!

OK, SO NOW I'M HOME.

I unload the car and put everything away. I'm embarrassed to say, I then retrieved the coffee maker I previously moved to the garage to remove the tempting visual from my sight.

I'm addicted.

Now it's GO-TIME!

The coffee's done, the 1st of 2 cups consumed, and the pick me up is just what the doctor (simulated doctor) ordered. With some necessary energy restored, I retrieve the bed linens from the dryer and get to making my bed. That's not an easy thing to do, by the way. Pillowcases, mattress protector, and the sheet's tucked corners... it's an exercise for the fingers for sure, but I got it done. It took some doing and it depleted some energy, so I have to head back for that second cup of coffee now.

ON TO THE NEXT TASK.

It's time to fill the birdbath and water the roses.

In my case, that means trucking a gallon pitcher of water through the house and out the front door no less than four times. And by the way, I repeat, it's too friggin' hot outside! I have a plan to clean my bathroom sink having already done the toilet a couple of days ago. There's absolutely no way to clean everything in a bathroom at one time – it's not in my MS capabilities. 'Work' triage is required. Everything has to be in fluid plans and performed in spurts, or else.

I HAVE TO LESSEN MY GOALS BASED ON MY ENERGY. SO, I refill all the toilet paper rolls in the holder thing-a-ma-bob, load a few items into the dishwasher, and sit back down to check my emails. The intended plan was to clean my bathroom sink, but I'm fading fast. I'll reassess that this afternoon. Well, I did write this story in the middle of all this, so I'm adding it to the accomplishments of my MS day.

When I think of what a hard day's work used to be pre-MS nightmare versus what it is now... it's a joke! Actually, I try not to think about that because it breaks my heart. I was perceived as a workaholic and I understand why they thought that. I genuinely adored my work and would love to be able to start it again.

I have to put that in context though.

TODAY, I WAS ABLE TO DO ALL THE THINGS I LISTED above, despite the daily challenges of living with MS.

SANDY O.

I'm doing good now.

'Stable' is the medical word for it.

I'm living an independent life despite this POS disease. I wonder if my ex-coworkers think that I have it good because I get to stay at home. The truth is, I think *they* have it good because they're at work doing important things. It tears at my heart like you would not believe. It's a crime to tell somebody with a beautiful voice to stop singing. I feel like that's basically what happened to me by medically retiring. I know that it is probably the smartest choice I've made for my health, and it did pan out in bettering my health, but like I said, it hurts, big time. It's years later and I'm still mourning the loss of my profession.

I PRAY FOR SOMETHING ALMOST EVERY NIGHT AND IN my heart, I know it's going to happen in my lifetime. I am speaking to a person who is not OK with failure.

Somebody out there… maybe you're reading my story.

You have an idea of a cure for this disease. Fight for us and have a full day every day in a relentless attempt to obliterate or prevent this disease. A US President inspired our nation to land on the moon with just his words.

TO THE INVENTOR OF THE CURE FOR MS, I THANK YOU in advance and I have true faith in you. We will shake hands someday.

It's time to land on the moon.

SANDY O.

17

MY PHONE DOES

JAN. 28

THAT'S a phrase I used to say at work when people gave me the sad look.

"How is your MS doing," they'd ask.

I'd say, "I don't have MS... my phone does."

They were used to my sarcasm and eventually got the point. I refuse to carry the weight of what this disease inflicts. It's just too much to keep ahold of.

When did that symptom begin?

How long did it last?

What was the intensity?

Screw that!

My iPhone will have to carry that bag of rocks around!

ANY TRIP TO THE ER OR A SPECIALTY CLINIC... THE nurse or doctor always starts with the same questions:

What medications and dosages are you on?

What's your medical conditions?

It's important to keep track of this information because often, what they have is not what's current. Always write down when you start something, when you end it and why – I mean that about symptoms and medicine. Just when you think you know your own story, somebody asks you a question that ties your brain in a knot.

ALL I HAVE TO DO IS SEARCH MY IPHONE'S NOTES FOR "medication" or "symptoms" ...and bada-bing, there's the current data at my fingertips. After the bit about the medicine, the usual follow-up question is if I have any allergies. Given the multiple medications and supplements I've been prescribed for various MS reasons, I have amassed quite a list of allergies and reactions to keep note of. Again, a quick search for the keyword "allergies" in my iPhone's notes, and all I have to do is say what I've annotated. The pictures you can take of your reactions help the doctors as well, and they're shown with the date and times taken. All your potentially forgotten recollections can be stored on your iPhone – it's one less heavy proverbial backpack to lug around.

I KNOW SO MANY PEOPLE WHO HAVE MS OR OTHER ailments but do not have smart phones. Believe me, my daughter had to convince me to get one a decade ago as I saw no need for it. It's taken me years to understand how beneficial this multi-application handheld computer is to my freedom. It was so stressful trying to keep track of the minutia of MS's antics... so I don't. No more trying to find paper tablets with often illegible handwriting. I simply jot it down in my iPhone's 'Notes' app.
- Dates of appointments and what was discussed
- ER trips and doctor's names
- When I was very fatigued

– When I felt like an extremely capable wonder woman today and why I think that

All these things and more are quickly stored in this handheld vault.

I USED TO WRITE DETAILED MS NOTES MULTIPLE times a day when I was at my worst. My goodness, I documented every damn body failure! I realized that I needed to change that from just MS documentations to significant events of all sorts. Once I stopped keeping notes of just the nefarious MS subject, the topics to keep note of broadened nicely. I added pleasantries such as, I adopted a dog, the hummingbirds are back, or I made a new friend today.

Life started presenting itself again.

My focused chronology of MS was fading to the background and in the foreground, was all the things life presents. I developed a new spectrum of purposeful and interesting notes.

IT'S ALSO OPENED ME UP TO FREEDOMS IN WRITING via the voice-to-text function. I wrote about that in a prior story, so I won't reiterate that miracle here. Ironically, back when I was working at a race car's pace, the iPhone became what I thought was convenient but turned out to be an arch nemesis in its proficiency. It literally robbed me of sleep that I never thought I really needed. Boy, did I learn that lesson the hard way! The single most significant and effective medicine I've ever had... is SLEEP!

EVEN NOW, HAVING LEARNED A LESSON TO PUT THE phone down before bed, proves its validity over and over again.

If I even look at the phone's brightness, it can prevent me from falling asleep and certainly invokes my restless legs.

Alas, it's a hard *drug,* to put the phone down. They're just so darned tempting!

I always want that last bit of news updates, to check my email one more time, or for my upcoming calendar reminders. That's another reason a smart phone works very well for our kind. It's so helpful to populate reminders or appointments into its calendar, and to modify how you're notified.

It's priceless!!!

So, THIS STORY IS TO CONVINCE THOSE WHO DO NOT understand the benefits of having a smart phone and how instrumental it can be to your stress relief and the regaining of your lost freedom. I'm sure Steve Jobs could not have known the amazing impact such a device can have for those of us with medical issues.

My shopping list, my to-do list, my appointments, my stories, my contact list, connectivity with others... Etc. This list can go on for days and I wouldn't be done explaining its benefits.

Don't be afraid of it.

I've had an iPhone for over a decade and I'm still learning how many things it can do for me. I no longer want to travel but can do so through my iPhone via FaceTime. Freedom by way of a handheld device...

WHO-DA-THUNK?

SANDY O.

18

PLEASE HEAR ME

FEB. 15

PLEASE READ this real story from a learning and helpful angle. My intent is not to hurt or offend anyone. My goal is for medical staff to learn something from it, and to empower the MSers (or their care partners), to be your best advocates.

TWICE, I'VE BEEN DIAGNOSED WITH TRIGEMINAL neuralgia, and both times, it was not the case. This was despite my professed, absolute knowledge of both painful originating events that caused it. My input was disregarded – a theme that unfortunately has repeated itself. The only results I see were my infliction of extreme pain and continued discounting of my knowledge of self.

My first occurrence happened in the late 80s. In error, a dentist was literally pulling a molar out instead of working on the scheduled task, which was to remove and re-adjust a tooth's band for my braces. He got distracted by a conversation in the hallway during that procedure and was literally pulling my tooth out! I leapt off the table in agony.

For 20 years, I suffered from recurring monthly pain in that tooth and its associated nerves. Because they could never see anything wrong on the X-rays, every year my repeated requests to pull that tooth was denied as they saw no anomalies in the images. The military does not just pull teeth – there has to be something wrong that they can see, given you are a deployable asset. Unnecessary procedures will not be performed, and they never could see that which I felt.

MORE THAN 20 YEARS LATER, I SAW MY CIVILIAN dentist and pleaded for him to extract this excruciating tooth. He wanted to look at fresh X-rays and I'm horrified, having already been through this, year after year. He, too, sees nothing wrong on the images.

Now, with tears pouring down my face, I say, "Give me the pliers and I'll do it myself!"

I was tired of decades of pain and it had to be done. Thank God, he obliged me and began the procedure.

His first tug drew his surprised response.

"Oh! It's cracked, and it's an old one."

Only a portion of the tooth came out with that first tug and he could see the decay in the crack. The second yank included the roots. They were porous from years, possibly decades, of infection. It looked like a sponge with divots – that's what my tooth's roots looked like.

I felt vindication from the realization that I had gone over 20 years with monthly pain (since a woman swells during her period), and they never could see what I felt.

The second very similar dental event happened and led to my second trigeminal neuralgia diagnosis.

I BELIEVE IT WAS 2018 WHEN I BIT DOWN INTO MY favorite sesame chicken from my favorite Asian restaurant.

Something was very wrong in that bite as it felt like deep-fried superglue immediately adhered to my teeth. In the back-and-forth jarring of my jaw, attempting to unstick that (*chicken?*) from my teeth, something was seriously damaged. Thank God, my food was to-go because what resulted was screaming from a mind-crushing, excruciating pain. A new word needs to be created because pain does not suffice.

I suffered horribly for days and finally relented to the ER. One glorious thing that was done for me to tide me over until the next day's referred dental appointment, was to give me one pill of hydrocodone. It removed my pain, and there was absolutely no wooziness, high, or impairment of any kind.

I was shocked!

What a beautiful medical advancement to relieve my pain and not impair me in any way. I want to stop for a minute and thank that ER doctor for his knowledge and administering of that amazing pill. I also want to thank the makers of that drug. Its affects were exactly... and I mean exactly, what my body needed – respite from the pain.

Now, I'm about as square a human being as you'll ever meet. I don't do drugs – never have. I don't drink alcohol or break the law. My only sin is that I swear too much. I do understand the liability fears doctors have when prescribing opioids now, given the new stringent laws. However, I am the last person on this planet at risk of being addicted to anything.

Well, Cheetos maybe...

Sorry, a little comic relief betwixt a heavy subject. To shorten this particular story, I will summarize.

I was given a three-day prescription of hydrocodone to let my body relax so I could specifically identify the culprit tooth or teeth.

Success!

I was able to ascertain the relative tooth's location and the process of scheduling a root canal started. They explained it would not be sooner than a month before the procedure and gave me a prescription for five days of hydrocodone.

Let's see...

5 days' worth of pills

30 days (at least) till the root canal?

That's math I can do, and it doesn't add up. The dentist had one other concern given my MS diagnosis – he was worried about the neurological implications and said I needed to see my neurologist ASAP.

I DID AND WAS QUICKLY DIAGNOSED WITH trigeminal neuralgia... again. I explained the circumstance and how the pain instantly emanated from biting into that *chicken*. The doctor pressed on and immediately prescribed me with medicine for seizures. He said that if the dosage didn't work, he'd amp it up to the tune in 4 separate times until it did. He was clear and stated this diagnosis explains the pain and also relates to multiple sclerosis. I was dumbfounded and seriously couldn't take any more conversations on the subject.

Here I am *again*?!

Everyone who has audible capabilities hears. How do I get my doctor to *listen* to what I'm saying? I was stuck in this vortex of my actual experience being bypassed again. I was so desperate to be heard – still am.

Shortly afterwards, I went back to the dentist I last saw and explained my dilemma. In that conversation, he said something that fit like a glove. People can take up to three months to recover from a traumatic dental accident.

Wow!

To know that there might be a resolution as simple as time was amazing to my ears.

. . .

I NEEDED TO UNDERSTAND THE NATURE OF THIS PAIN. For the next three or four weeks, I studied myself like a mechanical drawing – an electrical schematic of sorts. I had lightning rods of reverberating pulsations of pain that kept me in fear of any movement since the adrenaline caused more shocks and waves of electrocution. I couldn't talk, eat, drink, or brush my teeth and the pain basically had me bedridden. I needed to know how the pain was manifesting, what was causing its reverberations.

For fear of running out of the non-refillable pills, I figured I'd better start now. I never opened that hydrocodone bottle and haven't to this day. I needed the data of the unmasked raw pain to find the answers I needed. It's the troubleshooter in me.

I know, I know – bite your nose to spite your face.

When troubleshooting an anomaly, you don't try simultaneous resolutions because if successful, you can't ascertain which one made it work. Painkillers would mask that which I had to feel so I could figure out the beginnings, the agitations, the patterns of travel, and any resolutions I could sum up.

It literally took over 3 weeks for my body to overcome the nerve trauma that biting event caused, and my pain finally diminished to a more tolerable level. Even now, I cry remembering the intensity of what I went through. I knew that going from no pain (hydrocodone) to full pain (running out of pills), would've been harder for me to deal with. The root canal was finally done and for the most part, it was successful. The most important note is that it was not trigeminal neuralgia, which I knew... again.

The next subject is on my first MS disease modifying therapy (DMT).

. . .

HAVING BEEN GIVEN A GOOD RUNDOWN OF MY options in medications, I chose one. Soon after my 1st dose, I had my first round of hives. That side effect was clearly listed as a possibility for the DMT I was on. I brought it up repeatedly and showed pictures as proof. I also had several ER trips for it too. The physician's assistant (PA) expressed that I must not be taking the medication correctly or that I must not be drinking enough water.

That was not the case on either account.

I was doing the exact right thing and I reiterated that it is listed as a possible side effect for this drug. That same PA later told me to see an allergist despite my stating it happened within 24 hours of starting that drug.

I was referred to see an Allergist anyway.

Right away he says, "You know, this is listed as a known side effect for that drug."

I felt like an idiot.

"Yes, I've been stating that fact for well over a year," I said.

In an attempt to avert the hives, I was then put on three different medications – one of which I wound up allergic to as well. Returning to the PA, I reported what the allergist said about the hives being a possible side effect for the DMT. The PA gave me a snarky response.

"That's why he's an allergist and I specialize in MS."

I went through hell for years with recurrent burning and itching hives as well as taking three separate medications to try to overcome them.

YEARS LATER, MY BRILLIANT MS NEUROLOGIST (WHO has exceptionally, current knowledge), contacted his office to inform me to get off that drug ASAP! Apparently, I met all the risks for Progressive Multifocal Leukoencephalopathy (PML), which unfortunately puts the patient at risk of sudden death or an extreme debilitative state.

On to some of the risks:

Lymphocytes numbers below 800 for six months or more (I had those numbers for over a year)

My sex (F)

My age (50s)

I needed to be tested for a very popular common brain virus called the John Connors Virus (JCV).

I was tested and sure enough, I was positive!

Look it up – most of the population has it in the brain but it's not active or on, for lack of a better word. It's kind of like being HIV positive but you don't have aids. Having the antibodies for the John Connors Virus is not the same as being positive for the JCV. Positive means it's on and makes you more susceptible to PML, given several other factors. This is a good place to note that I am not a doctor or any certified medical person whatsoever. I am giving you the data I've found out from medical professionals as well as detailed research I've personally done and put into my own words.

So, I literally met all the risks for sudden death and had to get off my DMT ASAP. The prescribing office (not to be confused with the fact that I am the one who chose that drug), never tested me for the JC virus. Anyone with the antibodies can become positive at any time – it's not a one-time good deal blood test.

IN FACT, WHEN I BROUGHT THIS UP TO THE prescribing doctor, he was focused on another drug where the JC virus is a player (Tysabri). After explaining that new data is out there now since so many more people are on my DMT, it shows that the JC virus *is* a player with my prescribed drug too.

He said fine, do the research but it has to be from respected medical entities and gave me the ones he'd respect.

Talk about a mission...

I went to work on this big time!

Now hold on everyone, don't freak out that this doctor assigned a patient to do research. He already observed that I am insatiable in the fact-finding hunt, especially as it pertains to medicines I'm on. I also found this assignment showed me respect. He allowed me to provide the research to back the premise and I was actually complemented. For me, it showed he knew who his patient was, and I was doing the research anyway...

He and his patients may as well benefit from it.

I stirred my coffee with MS – I'm the perfect candidate to chase this rabbit, so off I go.

EXCLUDING ANY BLOGS, I STUCK TO RESPECTED medical websites. I certainly referred to the drug manufacturer's latest data and appeared a week later with a stack of documentation I highlighted affirming the new JC virus and PML risks. His reaction was to ask, what drug are you going on next? I told him I needed a break; I needed my lymphocytes to recover before I considered any more drug options. Some patients take over a year or maybe never to recover their lymphocytes count.

Further, something else happened when I stopped that drug. I've had absolutely NO allergic reactions – not one! By the way, I also stopped all the allergy medications at the same time as my DMT.

That means, all those pleas from me explaining that I'm allergic to this drug, as well as the subsequent allergy medicines I was put on to stop the hives was a shame – it was torture. I sure would've liked to of been wrong, but it turns out

I was unfortunately right and suffered for years with recurring hives.

THAT SAME PA ALSO ASSIGNED ME TO ONE OTHER drug that I'd previously been allergic to. Despite my warnings, they were disregarded as a fluke. The same happened with an ER doctor, despite my known allergic warning.

Yet again, I was found to be allergic to both drugs.

Yep, more bouts of hives and the same allergic reactions as previously documented. That PA nor the ER doctor ever acknowledged that my professed medical history was completely disregarded for years. More importantly, I was at a later appointment when it hit me to ask if the system showed an allergy to the DMT I stopped.

It did not!

That meant the PA never documented that fact, which means if I was ever incapacitated and wound up in that hospital, I could've been administered that same drug since there were no warnings of the allergy!

My informed warnings have been bypassed repeatedly and without justification. I'm not a stupid woman and I don't say things just to say things. This was different – my physical well-being was now in jeopardy. Before leaving that appointment, I had that doctor update my allergy list with that drug. I hate that I have all these examples, but I do. Believe me, I have plenty more, but they basically say the same thing – please listen to me.

YEARS AGO, WHILE ASKING ABOUT A DRUG'S SIDE effects as it related to my pre-existing condition, my doctor at the time said,

"And what did you get *your* Doctorate in?"

The inference being, do as I say.

I said, "I have a PhD in me, and I will always know more about what's going on in this body than you."

No doctor should be making a firm decision without hearing a patient's own history first. I've cried enough today with all the full recollections of these occurrences. There are so many more, but most wind up parked in the same unfortunate driveway. The medical community still has much to learn about patients.

Not patience, but PATIENTS.

How many others are out there and don't feel that they're allowed a voice?

I have a very big voice in defense of myself and others, and I have been repeatedly discounted of my own experiences.

What is happening to those without a voice?

I fear for them.

The pain and breaking of a human being have to stop. Change is required and updates to training curriculums are necessary. It's a tough story and certainly very difficult to write. I don't want some very good things to go unnoticed, because there is excellence in those same people I've talked about.

THANK YOU TO THE ER DOCTOR WHO GAVE ME THAT 1 hydrocodone pill that did EXACTLY what a pain pill is supposed to do.

THANK YOU TO THE DENTIST WHO GAVE ME THE BEST advice – that a dental injury and pain needed time to subside.

THANK YOU TO THE DENTIST THAT PULLED THE 20-year aching tooth and changed my life, and to the dentist who performed a root canal on that 2nd injury to relieve my pain.

. . .

THANK YOU TO MY FIRST NEUROLOGIST WHO ultimately learned who I was and respected what I had to say. I also thank you for helping me recognize when it was time to go through my work's exit door.

THANK YOU TO MY 2ND NEUROLOGIST WHO recognized my drive to work and pulled me out in the middle of what he found to be an MRI glowing significant relapse. I appreciate you figuring out that it would require a huge crowbar to get me away from work and into the hospital. Your competitive banter is always entertaining.

THANK YOU TO THE PA WHO HAD TO HEAR THE gruesome details of my symptomology and connected me to much needed support from a physical therapist, relevant prescriptions, and other support entities.

AND (NEVER START A SENTENCE WITH AND), A resounding thank you to the neurologist who specializes in this disease and unquestionably protected my life with that PML warning. Thank you for respecting my decisions and providing essential guidance and information. You Rock!!

SANDY O.

19

EXERCISES IN FUTALITY

FEB. 16

LET IT GO... Literally!

A SURE-FIRE WAY TO ADD TO THE FRUSTRATIONS OF diminished capabilities is to give it a headbutt (simulated). I thought about titling this story, 'Bastard Files', and explaining how the raw swiping of that large, rough file insists on the wood or that metal burr succumbing to its will. Don't get confused by what I just said. I don't mean you need to succumb to the will of MS – I mean you *are* the bastard file and can make some symptoms succumb to *your* will. The portion in the title about "*let it go*" is a new way of looking at and changing things that deplete your self-confidence via handicaps.

CASE IN POINT, I JUST WANT TO MAKE A SANDWICH and I definitely don't want to do the dishes. So, I reach for one paper plate and get another MS middle finger...

Denied!

My fingers will not let me separate one plate from 100.

I *am* the bastard file and will make this inanimate object succumb to my will. In the maintenance world, we called out the 10% rule. You need to be 10% smarter than the object you're removing/installing/repairing. It took me a while to figure out how easy overcoming this frequent frustration was. All I do is grab a bundle of paper plates and bend them all in half which jars their perfect alignment to each other. What remains is a discontinuity, a segregation between the plates that I can grab and claim my prize. I did it and almost happily leave the remaining scarred bundle knowing they will have to obey me next time, no matter what.

IT'S A THING.

I treat offending inanimate objects as an assailant that I refuse to let win. I think I wrote about this before, but since I just talked about the frustration of paper plates, this comes to mind again – tissue paper. One brand does this extremely irritating thing by taking the last bundle of tissues in a box and folding them in half. That creates an off-keister leveling of the box's whole contents. It interferes with the plucking of one tissue.

It's a guarantee that when that happens, every single box that I get will be ripped in half at the first denial of the attempted plucking of a tissue. I have boxes that I've cut down to half sized with their tops cut off. I place the contents of that ripped open box within them. Of course, I first unfold that last frustrating bundle and place it unfolded on the top (having to succumb to my will).

By the way, I do the same thing with coffee filters. With that, I wet my fingers and strum the grouping until one separates away from the others.

Moving right along, let's now discuss dealing with food.

. . .

ONE OF MY FAVORITE FOODS IS THE GREEN GODDESS salad from Panera Bread. Because I have adaptations when I eat, I tend to get my food to-go. I'd rather be in the comfort of my own home with the *isms* of eating than in public. I used to attempt the tossing of the wonderful green goddess salad with its dressing, using everything from tongs, a couple of forks, or a spoon and a fork. The frustration of never being able to do that minus remnants falling all over my counter added more tasks for me to do... i.e., cleaning!

This had to be overcome, so I dove right in... literally.

There are no utensils greater than the hands, so I dug my hands into the salad and folded it with that wonderful dressing. Talk about a commonsense approach – that is so much easier than the attempted finagling of utensils that never sufficed. Yeah sure, I get dressing all over my hands, but I have dogs who are waiting to assist in the process. I stick my 10 fingers out and they're ready for the cleanup (I'm laughing hysterically right now!). Of course, that's followed up by thoroughly washing my hands.

How-bout-that for a stubborn resolution?

My dogs are bonding with me via that delicious treat, and I instantly removed the stress of utensils getting on my last nerves! Remember, they are inanimate objects that I take vengeance out on. It's easier for me to wash my hands than it is to do the dishes.

Let's see... what else?

OH, THE MAIL!

There's entirely too much junk mail – we all suffer from that. However, I don't just throw it away as there are identity thief dumpster divers. I rip my personal data off the wasteful printed nuisance mail and later, I'll shred that portion. I don't know how society moved to this career of dealing with the relentless delivery of such garbage mail and fliers, but some companies have a sick joke going on. I can only assume they got with NASA for some space-aged glue because the opening of the envelopes is a ridiculous science project. I don't need to pick up a ton of anything with a dab of glue, so why are they using the same type of glue for a friggin' envelope?

Time for that bastard file mentality to make another appearance!

That little lip that you normally flip up to facilitate running your finger down the edge of an envelope to open it, is kiboshed. That nuclear adhesive won't let you do it! I will rip that whole thing apart and/or cut it with scissors along the entire length of the envelope. I only give it one attempt, and upon discovery that it's adhered via that excessive industrial glue, it's time to rip that puppy, half knowing I'm going to throw the irritating papers out anyways, so what's the loss? It's actually easier for me to rip off my individual information from the already torn in half envelope.

I'm not playing, y'all.

If an inanimate object is causing me that amount of frustration, I will win the fight every time. I am the bastard file!

So... what else can I touch on?

OK HOW ABOUT THIS?

It's often a physical endeavor doing grocery shopping as it depletes my energy. Thank goodness where I go, they bring the bags to my car which is a blessing given the shopping marathon I've just partaken in.

Now I'm home and sometimes, I repeat a frustrating mistake. I usually put my purse on, open my trunk, and retrieve and carry one bag to the locked door. The bundle of keys is in my hand, my purse is around my shoulders, and that clumsy bag is being lugged by my arms.

Remember, I'm already energy-depleted from the shopping trip, and I've just set myself up for failure by trying to do four things at the same time. I can't articulate the key ring bundle to the right key to unlock the door. I'm re-adjusting the purse out of my way, and the heavy bag in my arms. I'm getting frustrated trying to figure out what action I need to stop in lieu of unlocking the door. I'm trying to swing my purse behind me, relocate the bag on my hip, and having found the right key, now I'm trying to bulls-eye the key into the keyhole!

Flip!

My purse finds itself back in the way!

Ahhhh!

This is akin to watching the sand drain out of an hourglass. You know you have very little time left before you have to lay down, so you try to hurry to get everything done before the sand runs out.

FINALLY, MY BRAIN PROCESSES TO DROP EVERYTHING, pick up the keys by the one I need directionally, and unlock the friggin' door *already*!! I would rather have 1/2 a dozen eggs break having accomplished one thing, than have all the eggs intact having completed nothing.

I saw something decades ago that just came to mind – it was of a baboon trying to get a treat out of a hole in an earthen wall. I'm pretty sure this was on PBS – an experiment of some sort. A scientist put the baboon's preferred treat (I think it was a fig) in the hole, knowing it was only big enough for an opened baboon's hand to fit in. So, of course, in comes the first curious monkey, and his hand goes right in the hole for the delicious treat. The scientist intentionally added to the monkey's stress by walking up on it while its now treat clenched hand is in that hole.

The monkey freaks out!

It's flailing and screaming in a full-on panic. In its complete frustration, the baboon can't figure out that all he has to do is drop the fig, open its hand, and he could flee the scene.

Any wonder why that recollection just came to mind in the telling of the above story?

So, at least I figured out to drop the bag, fling the purse, and the keys to solve the problem. Eventually, I figured out to leave my car without my purse, without having opened the trunk, or retrieved a bag of groceries. All I have to do is carry the keys and unlock the door before executing any of those following steps. I still can't believe that I have to take things down to small increments like that, but it is the order of the day... every MS day!

IF I HAD A NICKEL FOR EVERY FRUSTRATING, monotonous item I've had to reconfigure due to MS's narcissistic intent, I'd be rich! You name it, I've done it. I don't dress the same, having ignored or donated anything that buttons up and replaced it with the ease of stretch choices in clothing.

You know, I'm going to stop there on the examples because I hope you get the point. I personally can get more frustrated than most people and have to... and I mean, HAVE to, figure out a less frustrating process. For those of you out there that can take frustrations with a grain of salt... hats off to ya.

I come wired for sound.

I simply MUST figure out a solution. The beauty of having a mind like that is that once you figure out one thing, you can easily parlay it to the next frustrating thing. In my psyche, I already know that debilitating things life throws my way are not to be succumbed to. It's a challenge I already know I have the answers to. Well, I may not have them right away, but I know I will figure them out.

I feel empowered and have felt that way since before my MS

diagnosis. I have my dad's ingenuity, and certainly his stubbornness. I know 1000% that God made me who I am and why I am this way. My job is to listen to Him and enact His plan. I am sure He doesn't want me taking the BS of MS... He knows my words have the potential to help those who are more easily overcome by challenges.

Yes, MS is standing in my view, but I have a mean right and I will knock that competitor out of my way and lay it out on the proverbial mat. As a result, my view is instantly restored.

You don't have to become me. In fact, I don't advise it. But I hope you gain some strength you didn't know you had and maybe open up your mind to devising possible solutions to things you we're told or perceived were permanent declinations.

Grab the reins and see if it's something that can be worked around, and/or rewired. I can't promise a cure, but I can absolutely tell you it will help empower you.

SANDY O.

MS – A LIFE DECONSTRUCTED

FEB. 17

I'M GOOD FOR 10... maybe 20
 Spurts it is – such is the new forced way
 Oblige I must ... or else
 No large containers, no bulk
 15 items or less, toilet paper for sure... but we won't get
into that
 Nothing heavy, or balance and energy seek revenge
 Wonder woman I was, careful and calculating I now must be
 Minuscule requirements only
 Voice to text iPhone dictation
 Scary news processing – coronavirus sickening updates
 Day 4... greasy pillow head
 Should I shower? Who will see me?
 My secret, she whispers
 Dogs are rambunctious today – bored of my stillness
 Shhh...I just want to write

SANDY O.

21

TIME TO EXTRICATE

FEB. 21

IF YOU HAVE NOT SERIOUSLY ANALYZED every single thing in your life that you can extricate in the name of your own health, I don't know what you're waiting for. Some things can mask themselves as essential pieces in your life. Work was just that for me as it was one of the sequencing numbers to my DNA.

For years, I kept physically declining, and coworkers would ask me why I don't just retire as they too saw what my body was trying to tell me for a very long time. Despite how much I loved something, it may not love me back.

Such was the case with my awesome career.

AFTER I RETIRED, IT TOOK ME AT LEAST A YEAR TO realize that I had to develop new normals minus the exodus from my beloved work. It's very much like that commercial of the guy at a café where he can't remember how to sip his coffee and winds up spilling it on his cheek. The commercial was about quitting smoking and learning to function without holding a cigarette.

So too is the physical, not just the mental piece of recovering after you've removed something so integral from your life. Yes, the mental piece of it is a big hurdle, but to land the fix, you must also deal with the physical.

I DIDN'T JUST LOSE MY WORK; I LOST A COMMUNITY OF like-minded focused individuals working on big solutions. In order to deal with the physical piece of all that, I had to self-flip a switch to start working on big solutions, but with MS. It's sort of like the railroad worker who flips the switch to redirect a train from one track to the other.

Serious hurdles were being thrown at me and certainly not when I expected them. At least for me, the surprises of afflictions made it harder to cope. You have to get over the shock of basically being flung a flaming bag of dog dung, before you figure out it needs to be picked up and the flames need to be squashed minus getting poop all over your shoes... metaphorically speaking of course.

So, in another story, I'd already talked about the fantastic help I got from a psychiatrist in facing all this, but now I want to talk about the specificity of the physical piece of it.

MY DAILY SOCIALIZATION WENT FROM DEALING WITH scores of people per day to basically zero. Getting over that loss physically, and in my case incrementally, meant I had to start reaching out to others who not only wanted to be there, but had gone through many of the same things themselves.

The MS support group I got involved in became a quid pro quo relationship. Not only could I get the socialization I needed, but I also got advice from people who'd been-there-done-that and had the answers I sought. As time went on and I was better able to tackle all things MS, I also found that I could provide the same for others in need.

THAT LAST PART HAPPENS TO BE AN INTEGRAL PART OF my make up. I don't know where I heard this before, but it went something like this:

If all you can feel or focus on is the injury on your hand, take a hammer to your toe and all of a sudden, your hand will no longer be your focus. Of course, that's not a sentence to be taken literally, it's meant to say that whatever negative thing has your attention, somebody else may have just had a proverbial hammer slammed to their toe and needs your help. You assisting that individual could be the refocus that makes your particular discomfort no longer your distraction. Good mothers already understand this premise.

If there's only one item of food left, of course you're going to give it to your child. Or, if you have no energy, you will, as soon as your child needs something.

Same, same.

ANOTHER IXNAY FOR ME WAS WHEN I GAVE UP SODA.

I extricated those 10 teaspoons of sugar in every 10 ounce can out of my life. To be fair, I really didn't drink a lot of soda but, I think I processed it in the same way a smoker puts a cigarette in-between their fingers... a habit.

What did I gain from doing that, and more importantly what did I lose from extracting it?

I really gained nothing but weight by drinking it, and I lost or removed a risk of having too much sugar in my diet and the potential for developing diabetes. I made a physical choice to extricate something that did not benefit me.

This next exodus was due to the fact that I did have to stop working. Every day, I looked into my closet for years and saw all the work clothes I could no longer wear.

Why was I torturing myself by repeatedly looking at who I no longer was?

It was also a facing of the fact that I couldn't even wear those clothes anymore with their buttons and zippers and whatnot. It was like I told myself every day...

"Yep, that's not you. You're not that capable woman anymore."

The solution hit me one day and it relates back to that socialization piece I spoke of earlier. I used to go to estate sales like scheduled calendar appointments, mapping them out to locations, dates and times. However, a lot of things changed with MS.

REQUIREMENTS AFFECT ME NEGATIVELY NOW, LIKE appointments or deadlines. So, I had to change my estate sale shopping to only if I ran into one in my normal drive somewhere.

In my neighborhood, I ran right by one and, as usual, began a dialogue with the woman onsite. The lady I was speaking to belonged to a church and explained that the sale of donated items benefited their outreach program.

Ding!

Right away I devised that my well-kept work clothes could benefit a bigger picture than me repeatedly looking in my closet and feeling pathetic. I filled my car with piles and piles of work clothes knowing that the proceeds would have a bigger purpose than my constant 'poor me' glances.

BTW, I'm still friends with that lovely lady today so how's that for doing two things at once!

. . .

ANOTHER STRONG IDIOSYNCRASY I ABSOLUTELY learned from my father is an extreme hatred of commercials and their over-accentuating tensile sounds.

Remember the big RCA TVs with the antennas on top?

My dad would tell us to turn the antenna to get a better picture. During those days, there were no remotes, but he had plenty of kids and if he heard a commercial, he'd yell:

"Turn it down, TURN it down, TURN IT DOWN!"

As we grew up, we didn't even have to be told because we too wanted the commercials turned all the way down – a learned behavior.

So, when I got up in the morning and made my oatmeal, the first normal thing to do was to turn the TV on and catch the news. Right away, I'm audibly attacked by shards of glass from the high-pitched squeals as if everything is so damn exciting in the ridiculous commercials.

It doesn't even matter if I mute them because the visuals are equally offensive in their flashing of circus lights and quick moving targets designed to intentionally catch your eyes! Even the so-called reporters and anchor people were so fake to look at with their completely modified bodies, voices, and fakery. They'd even smile during the reporting of murders and disasters. I can't possibly explain how absolutely disgusted any sighting of the TV had become.

For a while there, as soon as I saw there was a commercial on, I would turn the TV off countless times a day and couldn't get to the remote control fast enough! It always started my day off in the negative. I struggled with trying to find devices that could block commercials but never could. I finally decided that I would rather skip **everything** in the news, than hear one more overly excited torture of a commercial or broadcast! There's always the internet where I can pick and choose what stories I open. Having already suffered every single day with this audible and visual HELL for far too long, I finally cut cable.

Ohhhh Mmmmm Geeeee!

What the heck was I waiting for?

What an amazing stress reducer that simple act was, and I don't regret it one single bit. Oh, by the way, that decision helped my pocketbook too.

Next, there was another crucial extraction I had to do.

A BIG DECISION THAT PROVED ITSELF IMMEASURABLY beneficial to my health related to romance. My symptoms became so bad when I was still working, but even with all the debilitating problems I was going through, a realization kept presenting itself.

As it turns out, the more I overcame many of my MS limitations, the more the stress of *him* became clearer and clearer to me. In his relentless patterns of financial manipulation, of self-created emergencies, and certainly of his secrecy and double life, it was time to deal with the obvious.

My boyfriend's behavior and repeated bad choices were depleting my bank balance, my peace, and my health. His constant need for attention was disintegrating me more than my disease was. I chose to free myself from the stress of him. What resulted was the start of my recovery immediately and it still does to this day.

I'm not advising anyone to do what I've done, but I am advising everyone to consider that which causes you stress and to evaluate how it's affecting you. Out of all this, I know one thing... I know me. It feels right to be in my own space and to *not* have to deal with the antics of someone whose actions depleted me. I seek no vengeance and I wish no ill will. It pays me back nothing if things go south for him. However, our choices make our lives, and I had to make one that preserved mine.

To all the MSers, as you surpass insurmountable things with

this disease, always keep your stressors on your radar. Really study them and extricate any person or thing that is holding you back from blossoming again. You have a right to a good life filled with possibilities and good health. I wish you all peace and wellness.

SANDY O.

22

THE TEMPLATE

FEB. 26

I THOUGHT I was recovered from a lack of sleep the last couple of days but then there's the infamous Monday. I'm so drained, even standing up in the shower is a chore. My first task is outside trying to fix that which the dogs destroyed, but I can't stand upright. My knees are buckling. It feels like 500 pounds are pushing down on my shoulders and my legs are grossly affected.

First thoughts... Oh no, not again.

Second thoughts... But I've been here before.

THIS IS THE SUMMATION OF EVERYTHING I'VE written previously in this book. I'm gonna say it again... I have been here before. Any attempted fears, that *'awww geeeez, I'm getting worse'*, only got airtime for a fraction of a minute. I have had it where I can't stand, and the energy is just not there.

I told my then Doctor who ordered some lab work and ultimately prescribed me a B12 supplement. I'm not a big red meat eater so this is understandable but there's plenty of other ways to get B12. However, this supplement has worked for me when my levels are low. I don't take it very often, maybe once every couple of months and it reminds me that I haven't been eating naturally sourced B12 foods.

I'm certainly not going to tell you the dosage because that's a result of your lab results and a conversation between you and your doctor. What I am showing you is that once you find the answers or know that you *can* find answers, everything is solvable and/or understandable which makes coping with MS easier. Knowing those two words makes everything less scary.

Didn't I just say I slept horribly the last couple of nights?

So that equals an "**understanding**" of why my physicality is so bad today. B12 (for me), was also a rectifying "**solution**". I'm not freaking out because I couldn't stand fully upright for less than seconds.

I-have-been-here-before!

I now know things.

EVEN MAKING MY COFFEE AFTERWARDS WAS A FAILING experience as I couldn't stand without pushing my body off the counter (**cantilever**).

I know this algorithm!

Once you get into the pattern and figure out there's a B-side to that 45 record, you can take that **template** and apply it to the rest of your life.

Proof: The coffee is made; I sat for 15 minutes and began to feel the restoration I needed in my legs.

The Template works over and over again!

Fear not, MSers.

Go get your calculator and write your own algorithm. I'm simply trying to show you a different way forward – a hopeful way. My case is a successful way and one that I can count on. Scratch that, I don't count on an algorithm, I count on **me** having learned lessons the hard way.

. . .

IF YOU'RE NEW TO THIS DISEASE AND DO WHAT WE'VE probably all done by surfing the internet for what's coming down the pike, you'll see some horrifying things that are absolutely not true for everyone.

I think the first site I read said that you'll be in a wheelchair in 2 years, you'll have to stop driving, you'll stop working and blah blah blah...

Kiss my, you know what!

I'm telling you; you are your own internet site! So many are geared without hope or examples of overcoming. I've given you a few examples but now it's time to educate yourself. Help yourself even if that can only mean in your mind. Mindset can be your best or worst enemy.

IT'S YOUR BODY! TAKE POSSESSION OF IT AND CREATE your own template!

SANDY O.

23

CORONAVIRUS PREP'N, WHY NOT MS PREP'N?

FEB. 28

IF YOU'RE SITTING in a dark corner feeling sad, like it's all over, there may be proof that you're still alive and kicking!

I can't stop getting updates on the coronavirus. This world impacting sickness of a predictable virus spreading our way...

Why am I watching it?

Why do I need every single update?

Are you doing the same thing?

Have you gone out and bought extra water, canned or freeze-dried foods, extra vitamins and medications, etc.?

If you have done any of the above, you're still alive and kicking!

To hell with MS – this is bigger and your actions for survival are now on the table. I'm also seeing an awakening in my country that I'm very proud to see. In this whole coronavirus discovery, even I am finding out that we are literally dependent on another country for medical supplies and things like antibiotics! They also had ships turned around with cargo containing medical supplies like the N95 masks that the hospital staff and citizens need to stop the spread of this virus.

Since the news also reports that you can catch it through the eyes, goggles, gloves, and body suits are players too. It was reported that despite the shipment being already paid for, that relevant country literally turned that cargo ship around to head back for their own needs. I can't even blame them as I would've done the same thing to protect mine.

America, (politicians especially), you've got to be kidding me!

Who drew up any kind of bill or legislation that allowed the USA to be dependent on another country? There's diplomacy, but we should only be sampling in trade! Am I talking to myself here people?! That should've never happened, and I should've known that this was going on, but apparently, even those in the Senate and Congress shared in that surprise. There's diplomacy and then there's idiocrasy! We are an ingenious country – why else would the *elements* of the world be stealing our intellectual properties?

Regroup, people and country!

It's time to go back to self-sufficiency and use diplomacy as a sprinkling – not a necessity!

IF ANYONE OUT THERE THINKS I'M JUST TALKING about the coronavirus, you're dead wrong! The stories that follow will explain multiple hurdles MS threw at me – things that stopped me short of executing X, Y, and Z. While the subject of the story is a pandemic, it's also a pun for what you need to do so your ship doesn't get turned around on you. This is about what's necessary for YOU to proceed on and help you do as much as YOU can for yourself.

You may be bedridden, but you might be able to move an arm or a leg. Maybe it's just a finger, but it's movement. If you can, that is your daily exercise to beef up that capability (with your doctors' approval, of course).

Is your cognition well enough to think, and perhaps to at

least speak up for yourself? Can you tell somebody you're hungry, you're thirsty, or that you're in pain? Expressing those necessities is also a proverbial muscle you can flex. Practice speaking up for yourself if you can.

I know there's plenty of people out there with very serious limitations, but are you more aware of your limitations than you are of your capabilities? Not that I've ever done this, but I don't enter bikini contests as that's not who I am nor what I'm workin' with. However, as I speak into my iPhone and dictate this story, no string bikini was required. It is a capability I have right now and I'm flexin' it! The way I exercise this *muscle* is by doing it over and over again. Well, that and I always have lots to say.

Some MSers can order their food over the internet or call for a taxi to take them where they need to go. Some are capable of helping others (including animals), and some have to assist in their own care by voicing that they're in pain or the water's too hot in the shower, for instance. Doing the latter means you're involved in your own body, and that you're empowered or need to be. Expressing that to a doctor is necessary and makes you a warrior.

Grab onto the reins y'all, we're going for a ride!

I KNOW *I'M* NOT GONNA SIT BY AND WATCH MY CARGO ship get turned around without a fight. In case you haven't noticed, I'm kind of addicted to metaphors. Physical action is required to develop skills and/or re-wire things that are failing you, and to get you back into some sense of control and autonomy.

Back to the virus.

The news shows people in Wuhan literally being welded into their apartments – a forced quarantine. Yeah, it's probably necessary to stop the spread but what do you do once you become sick and are welded in?

The only thing you can do... fight!

Are you bolted in by this deteriorating disease? If somebody trapped me into an apartment and I couldn't get to the hospital when sick, the battering ram would come out! If MS had me sequestered to a corner of a room or a bed, the fight would commence.

You-are-a-fierce-warrior!

You may not think so, but I'm gonna ask you again...

Did you get extra water, given the patterns of store shelves being emptied that follow the coronavirus' country to country spread?

Did you grab some extra cans of food and meds?

I'm trying to prove to you that very unfortunate things such as this coronavirus outbreak should put a pucker factor in your backside and action is required for survival. Each time a dramatic stifling or hurling limitation confronts you, you should be adapting to the so-called language it speaks. Even in the collection of how I get updates and how it does not come from the standard TV channels is me fighting for survival. I'm looking at sites like YouTube's "Medcram" and "Timcast". There are many more, but that's just two. They pull from international papers as well as respected medical ones. I learned about the coronavirus as early as January 2020. I'm not an alarmist, but I insist on thorough information and am convinced you can't get that from one source anymore.

So, surfing I go.

I DO THE SAME THING WITH MS AS I TRY TO STAY abreast of new developments and research results. It keeps me at least knowledgeable of my options – even of my hopes. Just that one task is the flexing of another cranium *muscle*.

As I watch the spilling of this virus go from country to country and town to town, a theme shows itself. People want to survive, and they rush out to grocery stores to get the rations they know they will need, and suspect will run out. In an effort to slow the spread, the virus's originating country shut their whole nation down which means industry is not there to fill those shelves.

What's a person to do?

Well, I've certainly had my fair share of MREs while in the military, but I've never actually considered it as a civilian...until now. You better believe I ran out and got extra water, extra rations, first aid items, canned goods and so on. We only have to look at what's happening before we (meaning MSers and USA), can see what's coming. By that, of course, I'm talking about both scenarios – the progression of multiple sclerosis, and the emptying of those store's shelves (coronavirus).

For the first time ever, I see a circumstance that lends itself to a higher level of survival than I had yet been presented with. After much research, I ordered foods with longer shelf-life, freeze-dried foods and MRE foods for survival. Even if the virus never makes it to me, the food is good for years. It turns out that the freeze-dried industry is seeing 100 times their normal ordering now, more than ever before. That's proof that there are others out there that want to survive and who are looking at the numbers, knowing those grocery store shelves may not fill up. MS is designed to take necessities from you...

How are you going to fight that?

Like I said, my stories will show you some of my MS survival by way of fighting.

SOME OF MY STORIES WILL TALK ABOUT OVERCOMING obstacles but a plan has to be enacted. We all have a new hurdle

– the coronavirus spread. I enacted a new plan by stocking up necessities and hunkering down from the masses.

What hurdles are in front of you now?

Are you required to enact a new plan to get over the newest MS buffoonery?

America is resourceful, and so too should you be. I don't know about you, but I'm aiming for a life enjoyed.

Which way will you choose?

SANDY O.

24

IT BURNS MORE NOW
JULY 4

THE NEIGHBOR'S power went out – terrified.

Another stranded worm torching on the pavement – I can save this one...

And this one.

I look harder now.

I am the worm.

I *feel* that tortured child left in the car.

Cruel is too weak a word.

There are no words.

But I can't take it – MS won't let me.

78° and that is all... now.

Must have a backup plan.

Pushed off a cliff – old fear.

Car breaks down... June, July, August – new fear.

Heater's broken – winter... no problem.

But it's **June, July,** and **August.**

It targets the fair skinned me, the sun.

Vitamin D3 mandates it – but I can't take it.

Sunblock blocks it – Commando-Ish it is.

Only slices of sun – no more.

Water, water, and water... or else.

What do you mean, 'stand in line – outside'?

Details, I need details.

How far and is there AC?

No, thank you. I'll stay home.

Thoughts and fears boil me now – wish I was kidding.

Was that thunder? Wishful thinking...

This one's still wiggling on the scorching sidewalk – saved.

New first responder.

Every rescue saves me too.

I can't take it – WE can't take it.

I feel everyone's exposure now – every**thing**'s exposure.

None die on my watch *if I see it stranded* – I feel its singe.

I fear the singe.

The dogs, the dogs – they can't take it either.

No options – must devise the plan.

Must count down to winter.

My best friends = AC and winter.

Concentrate on the cold, Sandy!

Or else... the heat is hotter.

SANDY O.

25

ME CASA, ME CASA

JULY 16

YOUR KNOCKS WILL GO UNANSWERED. I don't want to buy anything. I don't care what you're selling, and if you're a neighbor, just call me first.

Such is my newly established and preferred survival technique of peace. I've talked about how I can't stand commercials and cut my cable as a result. I had to do the same with unnecessary outside stimuli.

My house is now my city.

Yeah, I still drive and yes, I still go to the store. And I'm a talker, so anywhere I go, rest assured, dialogue will be a huge part of it. I'm a fence talker and communicate with my neighbors, for sure, but once in my house... all bets are off.

I'm not a recluse by any means, but I don't like random people coming to my house, so I put a sign on the door. In effect it says:

'I don't wanna buy anything, I don't want to hear any of your pitches – I'm already saved, and if there's an emergency, call 911'.

Part of my MS learning curve equates to stress reductions for my health's sake. After all, if you want to build a house, it needs to come with plans. Engineering protocols have to be met and building supplies must be procured.

Me, in my space, is the foundation of *this* house.

I don't throw parties, there's no congregation of groups at my oasis, and my days are intentionally very predictable. In fact, I would hazard a guess and say it'd be 'boring' to anybody else on this planet. I need no more buffoonery afoot, so I control my environment.

MS AND ITS RANDOM MAYHEM ARE MORE THAN enough for me to juggle. My dogs thrive in this intentional low-key environment. If a squirrel has the *nerve* to walk teasingly in front of my back door, the 4-leggers invoke enough excitement for me, thank you very much.

In my world, who cares if I make my bed or not. Better yet, why does anybody make their bed? Perhaps for show, but I want my bed to be exactly opened for when I'm ready to collapse in it. Sleep takes priority in my world. It's the single most healing *medicine* I've ever been on and I give it anything it wants, and whenever it wants it. It's pretty much the only thing I've ever handed control over to – well, sort of. My bladder seems to call the shots too – obliging it, I must do.

The thermostat is part of the forensics to this crime scene. In my house, you could store meat in the winter. I keep the temp just shy of seeing my breath. I can dress for the cold, I can't for the heat... that is, without being arrested. Oh wait, I'm in my house so I'll just close the curtains and I'm all set (enter a flashing white light here).

There's another prudent reason for controlling my environment. Dear Lord, please keep the air conditioner functioning or else I'm done for. The dogs are now pampered to this particular temperature-controlled environment. Sometimes I have to make it even cooler for them than I need. They handle the winter just fine – it's the summer they get really distraught about.

AC... that's all I ask.

I don't demand much from the environment.

I like a small footprint on this world.

I STOPPED WAITING THE ABSORBENT AMOUNT OF TIME for my hot water to kick in. Now, I just put it in the microwave and warm it up. It's so much faster and less wasteful. I remember how irritating it was to hear the water run for so long, unnecessarily. I'll put an idea out there for somebody – go speed up this process to make the cold water turn warm faster so it isn't wasted. Sorry, giving you more ingredients on how this brain works. It's a problem and it needs to be solved. It just so happens that it's not my expertise... hint, hint...

Taggin' you in!

You see, when your brain works like this, you want solutions. Me self-containing in this safe place and orchestrating peace of mind is the solving of a problem. MS insists on stress reduction and it's not bargaining. Stress reduction is yet another reason I ask for assistance to lift this or move items from time to time. I have to recognize the things I can no longer do and allow people to assist me when necessary. That last bit was not an easy jump for me as a proud, independent woman.

MINUS THE DOG HAIR SEEMINGLY EVERYWHERE, MY home is the environment I insist on. The kitchen linoleum floor needs mopping – nope... not gonna do it. A wet slippery floor is a death sentence for an off balanced me. That's one good thing about this pandemic – Lysol wipes! Wiping up spots is something I can do. That's saving water and utilizing what I have with a purposeful use. It also helps me commencing with the exercise of bending and wiping the floor's spots. Today I'll clean my bathroom sink and perhaps my toilet. The shower is for another day – MS affords you shorter minutes to do nominal things.

All right, bits and pieces it is.

I will dust this shelf, maybe two.

Who's going to judge my efforts?

The other day, I took my strewn about pieces of local paper and commandeered my living room floor to put everything in wrapped-up order. Believe it or not, it took over an hour to do that one little task...

Bending, dates matching, folding, etc.

I'm so relieved nobody's asking me what I did today. I don't want to have to explain little nothings like that to anyone, but they are big somethings to me. My nominal problems were solved for the day per Sandy's house rules.

I CLOAKED MY BATHROOM WINDOW WITH A BLACK plastic portfolio because it makes sense. Why would they put silhouette viewable windows in the most private room in a house? I never understood that, but I damn sure fixed it! I don't even think about it anymore as I make my millionth trip to the most private room.

Moving on with the tales of my palace (*not*)...

I laugh a little when I get sent those weekly sales advertisements.

Clothes?

Ha, ha.

Why, I have all the pajamas I can use, and I use them every single day... pun intended.

I'm free from cloth at night and adorned with soft PJs in

the day.

My house, my rules.

It's not like I'm going to be answering the front door or anything! As long as I don't FaceTime, none would be the wiser. I mean, I do FaceTime with my family, but never when I'm in PJs or flashing streaks of bright white.

Day two, maybe day three – no shower.

And who am I insulting? Who am I disappointing? The dogs?

They stink so I'm pretty sure they don't care. I certainly haven't broken a sweat.

Ahh, home sweet home.

Milk... I love milk. I'm gonna have a big ole glass of it tonight and so the usual effervescence will commence. I'm lactose intolerant, but then again, I say, who cares? Who am I hurting... in *my* house? I'm not going anywhere today so I may as well enjoy that which my bones insist on. It saves on heating costs in the winter, *she says jokingly*. Unfortunately, the opposite isn't true despite having been occasionally called the ice princess.

The cooling costs persists.

BLUEBERRY OATMEAL/MIXED NUTS/SEEDS AND JUICE for breakfast...*again*, coffee and a blueberry muffin for lunch-ish, and a frozen entrée for dinner. That's my boring eating routine with spots of popcorn and squares of dark chocolate in-between. It didn't require me to get dressed, to do my hair, or put on make-up that I don't wear anyway. I'm pretty sure God knows the color he chose me to be – I'm surely not going to second-guess the Master. That's a schedule only a woman alone can appreciate. It's not scrumptious, but it's not bad and every ounce of it has a purpose that serves my body and reduces my stress. Remember, I don't cook!

It's not a leap for me to *not* be disappointed in somebody's expectations to fulfill some domesticated role I'm supposed to play.

Not so much... WhatEv's.

I can tell you that never works out despite my stark fair warning from the beginning. I will always be true to myself and will never fake a thing. I'm the wrong one. Since I stopped working, the only job I have to do is to place one foot in front of the other in this battle with MS's sci-fi intent. I don't do scary movies, and this is what I mean by being a skilled combatant to this disease.

THERE ARE DAYS WHERE I AM EXTREMELY PLEASED TO be stuck at home. MS wreaks havoc on your energy by way of fatigue, and there are instances of zero energy. I mean, you have to think about whether you *can* get up, not just whether you *should* get up. That's when I know my B12 is too low. I'm not a big meat eater; not that it's the only way to get B12 into your diet. In my case, one too many salads with not enough umph tossed in with it, plus a couple of nights with no rest equates to... *I got nothing left.* What better place to be than in the comfort of my own home when you're a blob on the couch? It's not a pretty sight but then, it's me, myself, and I as a witness.

In those times, I have to go back to the mindset of 'Mechanical Me'. **March,** you lazy slug.

Left, right, *left,* right, *left,* right.

The machine walks to get the breakfast. The machine lays tracks to the dispensing private room a million times a day.

The dogs have to go out and the dogs have to eat.

Who's going to check the mail?

The machine.

Fatigue is nothing I will tolerate for long because life does go on. If I'm going to get written up for not marching properly (simulated), it will not be in my own freakin' house – Me Casa.

SANDY O.

Get to Steppin', MS!

SANDY O.

26

MY EDEN

AUG. 1

As I lay here, comforted in the expectation of my words, this poem comes to mind:

MY EDEN

The cushioned carpet replaces the green grass of the original garden and comforts the sole of my feet.

The refrigerator's trees of options replace the forbidden fruit.

The polymer tall plants aligned in cadence in my paleo's view, blocking the neighbor's glassed Florida room.

My privacy is paramount.

From my eye's sight, it's green, green, and green.

I have plenty of walls, but not enough.

Pictures lie in wait for their turn on display.

My gardens hanging flowers...

They want their time in the light.

The perfect cerebral man walks the imaginary garden.

SANDY O.

He costs me nothing.
No competition with the thermostat.
My actual bed meets all my comforts.
The hum of silence is music to my psyche.
The hummingbirds are back for their Slurpee.
Sounds of fireworks muffled by pecan leaves...
Explosions of red, white and blue adorn my patriotic house.
I am one with my Country today... every day.
My welcomed guest...
She's saddened by the chaos...
Bruised by the inflictions...
Empathetic for the People's needs.
She was not designed for this.
She's mourning the loss of intent.
We are both in my house.
Independence with my house and Country.
God sees all – listen.
The Master Gardner blesses me.
My chosen Eden.

SANDY O.

27

WHERE I'M AT TODAY
JUNE 29

I KNOW you don't want to hear this but, I'm not well, as has been the case for the last few weeks. I'm in pain and never prepared for it. From the right-hand quadrant of my teeth/jaw, I continue to have this pain where it stops me from talking, moving my face, touching my cheek or chin, and it is accompanied by lightning bolts of debilitating pain.

You see, my gums keep swelling on the right side of my mouth and that's exactly where I had the injury from biting into what felt like deep fried superglue. I tried to make an appointment, but they said they're not taking appointments due to COVID-19. So, I have to figure out how to fix this.

Yes, it bothers me... scratch that, yes, it hurts me every time I have to eat, but it's especially hardest in the morning. When I eat, it's malleable food only as of right now. I can't grind my teeth. I think either an infection or gingivitis (new) may be at play here which agitates the same culprit, injured teeth. I've already adapted everything to tend to this spoiled child of a particular teeth pain. I have to microwave the water I *rinse* with (sort of), so it's not cold. I learned that the hard way, through many tears. I've switched to Sensodyne toothpaste in the hopes it will help. I dip my toothbrush in the warm water to prevent the shock of it touching my teeth. I pour my mouthwash in a small medicine cup, then immerse it into that warmed water before I attempt to *rinse* my mouth. I can't actually rinse my mouth because the physical movement of my cheek is so groundbreakingly painful. Even the simple unconscious lip piercing act of spitting is so intense, a lightning bolt of pain stops me dead in my tracks.

The dogs scatter from my screams. When it's this bad, I have to put a paper towel in my mouth to absorb my spit. There's something with the salivary gland that adds to this jolt that I can't explain.

Back to brushing, I have to move my head back-and-forth while keeping my face still. Of course, that has to be paired with grabbing onto the bathroom counter so as not to fall from such an intensity that it makes my knees buckle. There's no swishing when my teeth/nerves hurt this bad. I recently spoke to the endodontist's office who did my root canal, and she suspects there may be an infection in there.

I think she's right.

At least I had a couple of years of relief. Now I'll have to deal with the potential of an infection or gingivitis. More angles to the dangle, when I eat, I have to tilt my head to the left to keep food and drinks out of the cordoned right side of my mouth. I especially can't be outside in the heat and humidity because it raises my body temperature and causes swelling, none of which I can take, due to this condition – let alone MS. Any swelling is a recipe for a tortured existence. Advil's become an all-too-common ingredient for me now. There are several other adaptations I had to gravitate to.

. . .

It's not that I seek out the dark, it's just that for some reason the light affects me differently than most. It's not all the time, but I do need my house dark and don't tend to turn many lights on. I can't explain it but, bright lights seem to add to the acuteness of pain. I guess it's similar to you not wanting to be naked in a doctor's office with those bright white lights because you feel *out there* and vulnerable.

With pain, darkness has a calming ingredient that I prefer – that I need. I think this is a good time to explain the difference between an MS exacerbation and a relapse. A relapse is new damage, an exacerbation is the resurfacing of old nerve damage and symptomology. The latter of which could change what you are experiencing every day due to things like fighting an infection/sickness, being overstressed and lacking sleep, etc. There's a myriad of inducers that could bring back previous symptoms.

With that out of the way, I will continue on with today's state of health.

A couple of years ago, I had to stop drinking coffee due to the urgency of my neurogenic bladder. However, once I realized that I'm home anyway, the urgency of urination doesn't compare to the benefits of shrinking my blood vessels (my perception), and it does help my pain to dissipate some. This morning alone, while trying to eat my oatmeal, I was screaming and writhing in pain. I wound up collapsing necessarily onto my bed for more sleep. Even if all I was doing was sleeping, I wasn't experiencing the play-by-play of the darts being thrown at my jaw's nerves. That's part of the reason a lot of us sleep more, or in odd patterns.

You probably didn't catch this, but I just did something I did not want to do, but it has to be done.

. . .

I KNOW AT THE END OF A BOOK WITH THE descriptions I've just made within, everybody wants a Hollywood-style, clean and happy ending. After all, it's a heavy subject and we all want the person well in the end. I can't imagine anyone out there *not* wanting me to be OK, but that's just not the case today nor in the last few weeks. However, for me, there's a big difference between the then and the now of my symptomology. I know something for a fact that I did not know before.

In the beginning of the cascades MS threw at me, I thought it was all downhill from there. My walking started taking on the MS signature deficiencies and I had repeated bladder infections I had no idea I had, which caused a lot of my symptomology. When your body is already fighting the assault that is MS, any other infection that comes into the window disturbs your body's ability to fight the bigger monster – MS.

What I know now is the point of the book. Once you develop one fix and can associate that to other obstacles, you will be able to solve so many problems once you put your mind to it. There are absolutely no obstructions in front of you that can't be shoved out of your way, even if it's just a psychological adjustment. This is why this book is descriptively about MS, but at the same time, it's about everything and everyone. I'm just using the examples of my body to show you that you are stronger than you think you are. I'll lay it out with more current state stuff:

I'm weaker now, so less capable in my walking and normal everyday actions, but I know why.

THE PANDEMIC HAS TAKEN MY USUAL EXISTENCE AND shut it right down. In my virus avoidance, I've stayed in my house for the most part since the beginning of February 2020. I did everything right by stocking up in January for what I knew was coming this way. What I didn't do was prepare for the shutdown of my physicality due to being a vulnerable part of the susceptibility with COVID-19. I mostly stayed home and continue to do so through today. To write my own report card, I would get a C- with a need for improvement.

There's no reason I can't walk in the confines of my own house.

There's no reason I can't pop in the adaptive exercise video to make sure my movement capabilities continue.

I know that my current less-than capabilities are completely reversable by my own actions. I'm not fretting my current state because I know I personally can impact my outcome. I did not know that in the beginning. I thought every MS hiccup was another indicator of something completely lost to me. I was incorrect and had to completely change my perceptions. I just had to change my actions.

For instance, I've been going outside for very short snippets of time to be exposed to the sun so that my body can process vitamin D. I am no longer capable of trimming the bushes around my house. What I *am* capable of is taking a couple of snaps with those manual hedge clippers and when I take a couple of snaps, times a couple of weeks, I've completed the task my way. I'm not telling anyone to go cut their bushes. What I'm telling you is to reinvent the rules on how you do everything. Saved up pennies turns into a dollar, and the dollars turn into a 5er, and the fives into 10's... etc.

What I'm telling you is the measure of how you perform anything can be altered for success – even with MS.

It's not *less than*, it's just different than.

. . .

IN THIS BOOK'S LAST UPDATE, WHAT I'M NOT GOING TO let you have, is your way. I remember watching a movie once called, "No Country for Old Men".

What's wrong with that guy?

He's diabolical!

Who gets that way, how do they get that way, and surely the good guy's not going to be killed?

I needed justice in the end – I did not get my way.

I was tethered to the painful behaviors in that movie and finally realized the disturbing point. There really are things in life where you don't get your way. How are you going to handle those things? I cannot tell you I have all the answers because I don't. I'm just dropping some seeds, so they'll hopefully germinate for you.

The question is, will you water them?

As an example of how the flowers can grow, the following is a list of what I can do today.

It's now 4 or so hours after the timeframe when I was screaming in jaw/tooth pain. I slept for three more hours and then was able to shower and put my unruly, uncut hair up. I fed my dogs and let them outside, followed by the poop picker-upper detail. I was also able to drive to the store and walk to get creamer for my coffee. I prepared and carefully drank it. I was blessed enough to be able to *very carefully* brush my teeth using the procedure I've outlined above.

The pain is not gone, but how am I processing that?

It's not day by day, it's literally minute by minute. Even speaking this story inflicts random ice picks of pain you know where. Right now, some of the impairments I live with are that my balance is off, so I have to pay attention on how I walk. For 2 years now, I've been doing it without a cane or a walker. I have to be careful on turns because my body likes to keep going on a turn and I bang into things.

I'm bruised but surviving.

ONE BALANCE-RELATABLE DEFICIENCY WITH ME IS that you could poke a finger at me, and I would fall backwards. There's something about backwards where there's no equilibrium... It's dangerous which is why I wear an alert button, just in case. I still have burning pins and needles in my limbs, backside, and hands daily. They're predominant on my backside and down through my legs and the more raised my adrenaline is, the worse that condition gets. So, I constantly have to alternate from the seated position (with cushions), to the laying position. This is another reason I write with my iPhone and never sit behind a desk/computer anymore (not that my computer works).

Adrenaline can also affect my ocular physiology. If you cross the polarity of a battery, you have a force opposing the connection, much like what happens when you put a 9-volt's two leads on your tongue to check whether it's drained or not. It stings a bit if it's still charged. That's kind of what my eyes do when I'm under physical pressure – they oppose their own alignment. During that high exertion time, I found that if I squint my eyes like Clint Eastwood does, I can overcome that temporary issue. The part that I already know with that particular infliction is how short-lived it is. All I have to do is sit down in cool temps and within a minute, it's gone.

Remaining calm (which is not my nature), and reducing stress has a profound benefiting effect with MS. Continuing with my current state, the pandemic has limited my world significantly and while I'm a homebody, not being out there and doing things has affected my physicality and added to my anxiety. I suspect many of us are in that boat. I've also lost a lot of my muscle mass because my lifestyle's so different now.

I still deal with the sensation of boils and burning on my feet and calves but like a child's temper tantrum, you pay no mind. I do the same with symptoms as best I can. If my adrenaline and/or blood pressure is up, the pressure in my hands with the sensations of mini ice cream chunks of flesh missing... divots missing from my fingers resurfaces. At the same time, that adrenaline issue can affect my finite touch and the ability to pluck or separate little bits of something like paper plates, paper money, or plucking a tissue from the box. I often can't pick anything up, but, by golly, I sure can pick everything up.

Six of one, 1/2 dozen of the other.

I'd rather retrieve the bundle and return the remnants to the right place than walk away with nothing. It doesn't hurt, but it gets your attention, and you have to go back to life and ignore the brats of this disease.

My motor skills have declined during this COVID-19 sequestering time because I'm not doing as much, and that's my fault. I've also been writing a lot and that makes me more sedentary, so I know that's part of it too. All I have to do is resume my physical movement and exercising and that will jump right back.

Case in point, as my dad used to say, "Rigor Mortis has set in."

That's how he felt about his retirement and the stiffening effects on his body. Lately, I get the same thing with my legs stiffening up from lack of movement. That was the case the other day, so I got on my yard sale purchased, old incumbent exercise bike and went a few cerebral rounds around the neighborhood.

Problem solved... literally, and I'm not kidding, folks!

In my journey of MS's beginnings, I would think, 'Oh my gosh, I can't do this, and I can't do that'... but I know better now. My current mindset is that everything is recoverable. Usually, not *exactly* the way it was, but substantively it's recoverable.

. . .

WITH THE HELP OF AN ADVIL, MY TEETH AND NERVE pain diminished some and I was able to voice-to-text this story. I was also able to commence with necessary digestive activities (using the bathroom), which is often no small task with this neurogenic disease. Despite MS's mission, my cognition continues to be sharp.

Yesterday, I was able to unload my dishwasher and wipe down my kitchen counters. I'm physically sore today, but why? That's because the day before I was bending a lot, having swept my patio, which entailed moving minor items to get to the dirt. In a very rare move for me, I cooked my dinner. After resting, it took me twice as long to clean the mess than it did to cook it, but I did it and it was delicious. It's a very difficult thing for me to do and there was a lot of swearing and anxiety as a result.

This is why I don't cook!

Anxiety affects quite a few of us with MS. I'm sure it has a lot to do with the frustration of denials of function. It doesn't help that I was pushing myself that day. Still, it was my choice to cook, so I brought that stress onto myself. I also washed and folded a load of laundry, poured water for the birds and dogs, and helped others emotionally through some family issues.

Yes, my life has drastically changed in pretty much every way as it pertains to MS and its gaggle of affixed barnacles. I do not, however, concentrate or give light to the things that are different and/or changed forever. I am still doing, I am still living, and I am still learning to cope and probably always will. MS doesn't stop, so why should I? I want my last paragraph to be a peanut butter spread across this bread of life.

. . .

SANDY O.

Yes, the title depicts that this is a book about MS. However, if there's an obstacle in front of you whether you have a disease or not, the point of this book applies to you too.

This book can help you recalculate your brain waves into dealing with obstacles.

So, you didn't get that promotion, but were you close?

Are you now more informed on improvements you need to make for the next promotion time?

Are you now more trusted on the job?

Do people depend on your capabilities?

Did your car break down, or did good Samaritans appear to help you push it?

Did the storm damage your house, or is your family safe?

Is it too hot for you outside, or is your air-conditioner working well at home?

I can go on and on with what everyday life struggles are and show you that it's how you process what you're experiencing that can make or break you. It's your choice on how you look at what has *actually* happened. In my case, my learned lessons are due to God's timeline, not mine.

He knows when I'm ready.

Give yourself a break, examine your mindset, and if things are not working for you, affect changes to turn that around to preserve yourself. Do things differently for the same outcome. I'm not feeling great today, but every day is not today. It will be great again –

This I Know.

Jan 2021 UPDATE:

My tooth and jaw pain massively intensified for several months – evidenced by my loss of 25 pounds. I could not eat. I don't wish this experience on anyone, but I finally got an urgent appointment with the endodontist who did my root canal. The pain was so intense I couldn't even open my mouth to talk or put my mouth on the bite thing for a circular x-ray. The pain was profound. She did tests both to the tooth and gums and devised that it was Trigeminal Neuralgia. This is a very, very important point I hope everyone receives. Doctors will never live inside your body and you'll always have details they can't possibly know... but you do.

I WAS TASTING SOMETHING IN THE AIR AT MY HOUSE. Even though my carpeting looked immaculate, I would always immediately clean up any spot of spilt food or dog accidents with my shampooer... my old shampooer. Frustrated, my daughter did some shopping for me for a new shampooer and vacuum. Just one swipe of the new Hoover SMARTWASH carpet cleaner, brought up black soot-looking content despite having vacuumed and shampooed that spot before many times.

The old shampooer was not sucking up what it was putting down!

My goodness was the new one ever meeting that task! I attacked that carpet 5 times with the new shampooer using everything from bleach in the water, carpet shampoo, Febreze, and just plain hot water. Black soot looking liquids were coming up! The more I shampooed it, the lighter the liquids would become.

The shampooer did the trick!

What I was tasting all along was the sediment the old shampooer was not picking up. That dark matter was in my carpet. That sediment was literally being absorbed into my gums and teeth. Remember I had an injury in those teeth prior and by breathing in that foul smelling concoction, it was causing an infection in my mouth, gums, and teeth.

. . .

OBVIOUSLY, THE NEW VACUUM AND SHAMPOOER WERE extremely pivotal to stopping the smell/taste and picking up that dark fowl liquid. For me, that wasn't enough. To be on the safe side, I went ahead and had my entire house's carpeting replaced. Here I am, months later, and the smell and taste are gone. For clarification though, as they were removing the carpet there was no sign of mold – it was all in the surface of the carpet and the shampooer took care of that.

Fast forward, I'm at an appointment with my neurologist. He, too, agreed it was not trigeminal neuralgia because Advil would have no effect on trigeminal neuralgia. I have been saved by a new shampooer, a new vacuum, and my choice to replace my carpeting. Since then, I have very minor instances of pain that have to do with that biting culprit tooth, but nothing, and I mean nothing, as debilitating as what I was going through when I tasted the sedimentary remnants of what was in that carpet.

So, here's the question:

How in the world is a doctor supposed to know this level of detail of what I'm going through with my carpet, something I hadn't even figured out at that time?

It's impossible.

THE ENDODONTIST'S DIAGNOSIS OF TRIGEMINAL neuralgia made complete sense given my symptomology at that time. She could not have known the backstory to what I was experiencing at my house. This is what I mean by a doctor cannot know the full story – you are in the body. It's not their fault – they're trying to help, and it's not my fault that I have to dismantle everything to get to the root cause. It cost me an arm and a leg to replace my carpeting, but I am not in debilitating pain anymore!

Problem solved the hard way... and I mean, the HARD WAY! In my case, it was through months of pain.

It's a happy ending, y'all.

Always be in charge of your body and it's perfectly OK to insist on what you know or are experiencing.

SANDY O.

28

SIGHT VS VISION

JULY 6

As I've said previously, I have Relapsing Remitting Multiple Sclerosis and right now, there is no cure. I see what's in front of me and I cannot deny it's progressive nature.

That's Sight.

Everything within me predicts a cure will be found in my lifetime. Certainly, more disease modifying therapy options will be developed and they'll get closer to addressing many of the current potential side effects.

That, my friends, is called Vision.

When I carefully place my oddly gaited steps on the pavement, I am using my sight. When I look at my future, I am steeped in the vision and confidence of so much progress I see happening to combat this disease. I know they're getting closer to being able to repair the nerve's protective myelin sheath that gets damaged in the process of this disease. One step away from repair is to restore.

How can I succumb to defeat with such promising efforts being done by the smart ones, the dedicated ones?

Thank you for all those who are gravitated to these honorable endeavors such as this.

Defeat?

No, thank you. I'll stick to the vision for how I'll gauge my future.

I AM CERTAIN TO MAKE PLENTY OF LOGICAL DECISIONS that will make my life easier. They're moving quickly with advancements in smart homes that will allow for longer independent living. Highlighting the positives is something I'll never hesitate to announce and/or be embarrassed of. If the cure comes after my progression puts me in a wheelchair, for instance, I will have the most bad-ass wheelchair you've ever seen and leave tracks everywhere I go... and I will go! The mobility options with Uber's and the like are another positive to overlook a negative.

Given my current state of mobility, I don't see a wheelchair in my near future but then, God has the master plan, not me and it's my job to listen. Sometimes he has to rack his knuckles on his holy table to get my attention, but I'm getting better at hearing him the first time. I know it's through his direction that I am finding so many of the get-around avenues to what this disease tries to stop me from doing. The prior stories depict plenty of that. He's touching the brains of those who can figure out natural fixes to MS's deficiencies.

Movement, repetition, nifty devices to assist, and let's not forget determination. Even medical trials with a negative result are still telling them something usable. The results streamline the playing fields of potentials.

BEFORE MY FIRST SUCCESSFUL OVERTAKING OF THAT which afforded me *nothing* good with this disease, all I saw was what I could not do. Crack an egg successfully, being denied the security of just walking without falling, or an inability to use the restroom was a blatant withholding of my normality. My vision is far stronger than this disease's intentions are.

All the things I just mentioned, I've prevailed over. It's my sight that recognizes when I'm in extreme fatigue and glued to my couch or bed, but my vision takes the lead with a plan to overcome. If you ever run out of ideas, the MS surfing field is plentiful.

I go to several.

One in particular is MSworld.org. I look at their "MS in the news" for the latest and greatest on several studies. They have a conference center where I can watch MS conferences and never leave the comfort of my own home. They also have an awesome chat room – the whole thing is run by and infiltrated with us! We MS'ers are the ones in the chat room asking and answering questions to each other. This community is profoundly capable of telling you what they've learned that works for them. Of course, none of that forgoes your conversations with your own doctor, but it's a great community to experience. I remember when I had to stop working and lost the sea of people I was used to talking with. I found that chat room and it fed an emptiness I didn't even realize I had. People have answers and people have problems. On any given day, you're going to be on one side or the other of that fence. They'll not only have answers for you, but you'll also have answers for them, the more MS savvy you get.

Even if it's by way of what you've found on reputable sites and are spreading that word, or from some successes you've had personally, you'll benefit from the exchange. That same site also has an entire category (Abilities Expo), for what's new in your options with assistive devices. You might be suffering from something, thinking, 'That's it I'm done... it's all done', but there might be something out there that can be of assistance to you. There's so much positive news out there. Heck, this morning I just read an article through the national multiple sclerosis society of a promising result in mice where motor learning is repairing the myelin sheath.

I'VE PERSONALLY HAD THE PLEASURE OF ATTENDING gatherings and day seminars where the lessons are with me every day (thank you to the national multiple sclerosis society [nationalmssociety.org], cando-MS.org, and others).

Please don't underestimate the help that is out there. I know I'm repeating myself in this book, but it's with good reason. Never beat yourself up for repeating good things. Every nail needs a few good whacks from the hammer to properly set. Think of it as a mature lady telling everybody that she's now a grandma and to look at these pictures. I'm happy to be repeating good news. I'm just showing you the pictures, y'all!

The smallest success you'll have from an attempt to recover from anything will have a magnification factor that will open up your world! It's the power of knowing what you know.

Let's make the word of the day, "recoverable". If you're sad, if you're hurting, or if you have no vision for your future, I'm here to tell you what's on the other side of defeat's door. The sky is so blue, nature's greens will consume you, and you will begin to appreciate all the things you could not see behind the door of defeat.

Push the darned door open, friends!

Chin up because the good stuff's out there. You just have to focus your lenses, i.e., "calibrated eyes", to see it.

To show you that it works, I'm gonna leave you with a list of some of the things I couldn't do, but now can (✔ = solved):

1. Had to use cane and/or walker ✔
2. Shower with shower chair ✔
3. Drunk like slurred speech ✔

4. Cloudy cognition ✔
5. Hold an instrument like a pen, a fork, or use a toothbrush ✔
6. Put my shoes and socks on ✔
7. Get dressed ✔
8. Unable to put my hair up ✔
9. Go #1 or #2 ✔
10. See straight (due to optic neuritis or esotropia) ✔
11. Drive ✔
12. Sleep ✔
13. Put my fingers together like the number four ✔
14. Walk heel to toe ✔
15. Run the heel of 1 foot down the shin of the other leg ✔
16. Fell up to 10 times / day ✔
17. Handwrite ✔
18. Bend down ✔
19. Get up from a seated position unassisted ✔
20. Cook (if I need to) ✔
21. Open jars and containers ✔
22. Write a check/pay my bills ✔
23. Wash the dishes ✔
24. Replace my bed linens ✔
25. Wash and fold loads of laundry ✔

SOMEBODY, STOP ME!

That's just a fraction of the things that I've been able to overcome. Not all of the things listed above I can do every day nor all the time, and it's by no means all-inclusive of what I've overcome. It's also not encompassing all the things I still cannot do, some of which I've either let go of or put off for another day to tackle.

In my opinion, it helps to remember that when you get hit with massive symptoms, the best way to deal with them is to literally peel back the circumstances involved so that you can get to, 'Oh, now I understand', as soon as possible.

For instance, it's criminally hot today. My body is particularly affected and under high temps. I wind up moving like a toddler learning to walk with their hands out for balance. That's how severely affected by heat I am. The weather is supposed to get even worse in the next couple days, so I know the clock is ticking and I have to make a couple of trips. I intended to visit one store, but it turned into four in my search for Lysol wipes. Since I only shop within 3 miles of my house, I'm never gone for long. However, it's about 500° outside right now – that was a kick in the pants for this MS patient for sure.

IN TODAY'S HUNT, I FOUND ANOTHER BRAND OF disinfectant wipes called NICE and picked up a few other things I needed. Still needing dog food, I pressed on to the appropriate store. Remember, it's still 500° outside and every time I leave my car or a store, the temperature sledgehammers me bigtime! I got home and only unloaded the freezer stuff that I bought, literally succumbing to my weakness on the couch.

I'm spent!

There's no denying that I just basically got my butt kicked for a few short trips that took no more than 45 minutes, collectively. What I know now is that all it will take is a few minutes in the AC and laying down, and I'll be back up and at it again.

I didn't know that in the beginning. I was stuck on the *sight* of what was happening to me. I used to hone in on the fact that my body is shutting down, and poor me. What I absolutely know now is that my body *has* to rest and recover – there's no way around it.

I want to show you the rawness of when I was in the very beginnings of solving problems and still distracted with my odd symptomology. This would've been a timeframe where I was just getting started with the focusing on solutions.

This is from my MS diary entry three years ago:

"JUL 4"

"THE BULLSHIT WITH MY HANDS REMAINS. DEXTERITY AND THE switching, flipping, turning of anything is not there and, in fact, when I do those things, it tends to fall off the top of my hands and I can't grab it. I could still grab strongly but when I don't tell my body to do it, like when I'm walking or something, my hands are completely laid out like a paralyzed person's and my arms drag along with it.

Things that are difficult are the grabbing of my toilet paper. I could feel it but the grabbing of it is affected. The holding and articulation of a pencil or pen to write is still jacked up. Keeping ahold of or turning my remote around in my hand is limited. Picking up of any one thing pisses me off because I go to grab one thing and I wind up grabbing a whole wad of things with it. I can feel the difference and find sensation, but the grasp will take the whole pile instead of the one thing.

The same effect goes for when I walk.

If I don't think about each step then it's very labored, weak, and unbalanced. But, when I tell my legs, 'Do what the hell I say', and concentrate on it and only it, I can do the action so much better. But boy, is that process exhausting. I did definitely feel the fake boils sensation on my feet today which I don't remember being strong enough to feel the fake boils like I did today. Ironically, both the strong pins and needles throughout my arms, hands, butt, legs, and feet are greatly diminished when I lay down and rest. However, when I lay down and rest, I am so much weaker and feel more imbalanced when I do get up."

. . .

THE ABOVE SNIPPET FROM MY MS DIARY SHOWS MY fears back then, but at least I'm realizing some things and enacting plans. You can see my frustrations of not knowing what on earth was happening to me. You can also tell from what I wrote that it was the beginning of that story I wrote in this book, "Mechanical Me".

I have five years of extensive diary entries that are even shocking for me to read. There was nothing easy about the timeframe when I was being bombarded by symptom after symptom. I don't remember how long it took me to get to the point of starting to visualize solutions but, the quicker you realize this, the faster your recovery will be, both physically and mentally. Use your visual sight for tending to the handicaps of the day but use your **VISION** for your view of the future.

What am I going to do tomorrow?

What bird will make an appearance today?

I can't wait for winter to get here, and it will get here. My vision tells me so and I look forward to it.

I hate the hot days of summer.

I was trapped in my body for 10 minutes today from the heat. I laid there and recovered, and then I fed the birds and gave them water. I am now sipping the coffee I prepared as I write these words.

The future is bright if you use your **VISION**.

Come join me.

SANDY O.

ACKNOWLEDGMENTS

My first heartfelt acknowledgment goes to the Arbuckle Publishing House team. Kayla and Elle were so receptive and respectful of my need to retain my voice and experience with this disease in this book. Their staff artist, Nicole, is profoundly talented. Her work and perspective of my vision communicated so many of the elements I could've never realized. Her exceptional cover depicts the points my book is trying to communicate beautifully. I'm so honored to have worked with the exceptional APH team.

Thank you.

I'd also like to thank my MS support group who have seen me through some of the darkest times with this disease. They were the ones that put my name in for an educational seminar held by the National Multiple Sclerosis Society (NMSS). That weekend was my watershed moment. It was in that seminar that I learned so much that taught me to take my very qualified critical eyes and redirect their gaze to the problem-solving of my own MS symptomology.

Additionally, the MSCan-Do organization has been

instrumental in my positive outlook as well as providing helpful tricks to get around MS's hurdles. My MS journey has also been so positively affected by the MS World Organization. They helped me realize that I am not alone in this fight with their wonderful community of like-afflicted participants. Both their informative news and the fact that they gave me a voice greatly impacted my vision for the future. Their MS community is exceptional, both as a learning tool and as a camaraderie amongst all of us experiencing MS.

Lastly, I'm so proud of my daughter who stepped in to help me during a critical time. I know a lot of this disease is scary, certainly to the onlooker, however, she saw me through an injury that I am so incredibly thankful for. I also want to tip my hat to friends and family who've heard some of these stories that I was compelled to write. Being heard became a necessity for me and they were there – ears on tow.

My last thank you is to many of the medical staff which my stories will outline in detail. I'm a person who can fix many things but was humbled to see how many people knew far more than I did and helped me far more than I could. All your kick starter help stays with me to this day. You all rock and are owed a resounding, THANK YOU! You're all genuinely appreciated and sadly, underappreciated.

ABOUT THE AUTHOR

Sandy O. was born in a large city but currently resides in tornado alley. With an eclectic background, Sandy's career had her living and working globally. That experience added to her admiration for her country and love for the differences in people and cultures. She seeks no fame but being of good purpose is a part of her make up. God bestowed Sandy with the tenacity to view nefarious obstacles as speed bumps that she will overcome. Her only addiction is metaphors which is perfect for somebody that has a lot to say. Sandy believes that there's nobody on this planet that she can't learn something from.

CPSIA information can be obtained
at www.ICGtesting.com
Printed in the USA
LVHW090008180521
687462LV00030B/350/J